COLLECTION MANAGEMENT

against
the grain

Other Books by Diane Kochilas

MEZE

THE GLORIOUS FOODS OF GREECE

THE GREEK VEGETARIAN

THE FOOD AND WINE OF GREECE

against the grain

150 Good Carb
Mediterranean Recipes

DIANE KOCHILAS

wm

WILLIAM MORROW

An Imprint of HarperCollinsPublishers

FIRST EDITION

Printed on acid-free paper

Library of Congress Cataloging-in-Publication Data
Kochilas, Diane.
    Against the grain : 150 good carb Mediterranean recipes / Diane Kochilas.
      p.   cm.
    Includes index.
    ISBN 0-06-072679-2
    1. Reducing diets—Recipes.   2. Cookery, Mediterranean.   I. Title.
RM222.2.K575   2005
641.5'635—dc22

641.5635

2004060904

05 06 07 WBC/RRD 10 9 8 7 6 5 4 3 2 1

For Yiorgos, Kyveli,
and the big V, with love

Contents

Acknowledgments

THIS BOOK CAME ABOUT AFTER AN ATKINS DIET STINT AND DUR-
ing a conversation with my agent, Doe Coover, who first broached
the idea to me. Thanks, Doe, for encouraging me. I owe thanks to
Harriet Bell, my editor at William Morrow, who is both unsparing
and caring, exactly the two traits every writer needs in an editor,
and I have enjoyed working with her over the years. I owe great
thanks, too, to my organized, earnest friend Brigitte Bernhard Fat-
sio, who came as a godsend into my kitchen almost a decade ago and
helped me test and retest the recipes in these pages. I want to thank
Teo, too, for being a good sport and trying everything. Patty San-
telli aided tremendously with the nutritional counts, running and
returning the recipes, making suggestions on where to cut back on
fat and carbs, and doing so from a distance of many miles with
cheerfulness. Thanks.

I owe a million thanks to Christos Valtsoglou, Achilles Perry, and Michael Parlamis, owners of Pylos restaurant in New York City, for which I am a kind of chef by proxy, arriving on their doorstep a few times a year to do special events and new menus. More than a few of the dishes in these pages derive from those long hours in their East Village kitchen. Since this book was worked out mostly in my own kitchen in Athens, Greece, as a recipe-driven project, I want to thank a few friends who have been generous with their products. Mainly I want to thank Aris Kefalogiannis and Dimitris Paraskevopoulos, owners of Gaea Foods, for the olives and tapenades, but above all for the endless river of their excellent Greek appellation olive oil that flows in my kitchen at all times.

Books always are born thanks to a certain degree of sacrifice, usually of one's time. In my case, that's time away from my family, time spent buried in a computer screen or over a pot of food or on one or another countless forays to supermarkets, farmers' markets, fish markets, and the like. Last but never least, I want to thank my family—Vassilis Stenos, Kyveli, and Yiorgos and the whole gang on the other side, Koko, Nia, George, Tom, Kris, Katherine, Paul, Trif, and Zoe. They always stand by me and I am thankful for that most of all.

against the grain

Introduction

SEVERAL YEARS AGO, AFTER JUMP-STARTING MY OWN DE-
sire to shed the pounds I put on during pregnancy, I went
on the Atkins Diet. I soon realized that I was feeling great,
so much less bloated, and so energized, by eating a diet high in protein but low in carbohydrates.

To accommodate my own palate and body temperament, I
curbed some of the fat that is egregious on Atkins, albeit the cheeses
of the Mediterranean, especially those of Italy, France, Spain, and
Greece, are a constant source of both inspiration and temptation. I
began to rethink the foods I have always loved to cook, dishes rooted
in Mediterranean traditions that are based on fresh, seasonal vegetables, chicken and other poultry, some red meat, and lots of fish
and seafood. After enduring the two-week carbohydrate abstention
period that the Atkins diet and all low-carb diets require, and last-
ing through phase one of Atkins for another few weeks, I started to

miss some of the soul-warming dishes that are part of the food traditions in the Mediterranean, dishes such as a steaming plate of pasta, soothing rice, and, of course, bread. I could not imagine the rest of my life without ever again enjoying these basic comfort foods. So they slowly crept back into my diet, and so did the weight.

I tried again and lost again and gained again several times before realizing that I was rejecting what seemed most reasonable and wise. I should have listened to one of the basic tenets of the Mediterranean diet and of the Mediterranean lifestyle in general, that moderation is the key to health, that nothing should be had or done in excess.

Right about then, the South Beach Diet became wildly popular. The diet makes sense because it recognizes the importance of a well-rounded diet, yet it takes into account what I like to call the human foible element, the realization that no matter how much discipline one has it is virtually impossible to endure a diet that forbids some of the world's most pleasurable foods. Instead, South Beach seemed to adhere to the nothing-in-excess tenet. After the initial phase, pulses, legumes, and some grains are slowly allowed back on the table. But they are always in whole form: whole wheat and other whole grain breads, brown or wild rice, even whole-wheat pasta. I liked that.

By now it is well known that the low-fat craze that gripped the country and provided a field day for food manufacturers actually helped spur the American population toward record-high obesity levels. Likewise, the complete anathema so many people began to feel toward common, everyday foods, such as bread, verged for a while on hysteria. What has been missing on the food front for a long time is plain old common sense. Americans' obsession with time and speed has also added its own dimension to the dinner table. Not only does food have to be devoid of fat, or, worse, imbued with fake fat, or, now, devoid of carbs, it also has to be prepared in record time.

The food industry inevitably responds with an all-out assault on whatever is the fear of the day. For decades now Americans have been caught in a vicious cycle, on the one hand victimized by aggressively aggrandized food fears (advertising does that) and then, on the other, pacified with a magic pill: fake fats that let you eat all you can, low-fat, high-carb processed junk that delivered nothing but an obesity epidemic and all the diet-related diseases that come with it. I can't help but feel that the litany of processed low-carb products prey on those same fears.

My idea of dinner is to spend time actually cooking it, not just assembling various components and popping them into a microwave. I never set out to write a diet book, and this is not a diet book. Instead I set out to develop dishes that fit within my own Mediterranean sensibilities but that also helped me keep my resolve to eat real food that could easily fit into the second and third phases of diets like South Beach.

The key to finding a balance between the body's need for energy (carbohydrates) and the excesses of any high-carb diet is to follow that age-old Mediterranean tenet: nothing in excess. That is what South Beach more or less proclaims, that there are, in other words, good fats and bad fats and good carbs and bad carbs. That's what makes it so appealing. The fire-and-brimstone approach to dieting can only result in a fall from Grace.

I always knew instinctively that the Mediterranean table was inherently healthful, yet I always gained weight when I indulged in pizza, pasta, risotto, couscous, and—my weakness—baked potatoes dressed with olive oil and coarse salt. The Mediterranean table without pizza, pasta, rice, or bread might seem brutally devoid of all the things most people love about the region's many cuisines.

Low-carb Mediterranean cooking might seem like an oxymoron, but good-carb Mediterranean cooking certainly is not. The very words "Mediterranean Diet" bring to mind the carb-heavy dietary pyramid and the important role that grains—especially wheat and rice—as well as other carbohydrate-laden foods, such as pulses and legumes, play on traditional tables, from Turkey to Spain.

The traditional diets of the Mediterranean have always relied more on vegetables, pulses, and whole grains than on excessive quantities of protein. In many regions of the Mediterranean, white flour was, ironically, a luxury to be enjoyed by the wealthy, and by the masses but once or twice a year. In Greece, for example, fluffy, nutritionally vacuous white bread is still called "luxury" bread. Dark, wholesome, whole-grain bread was cheaper and considered inferior. It took decades for that error of judgment to be redressed. In this book, the use of grains is fairly limited to a few brown rice dishes, one recipe with wild rice, and some barley bread. Whole-wheat flour appears here and there in a few dishes. On the other hand, legumes and pulses such as lentils, white beans, chickpeas, and black-eyed peas are among the foods I love most, and they appear in carb-count-friendly proportions in several recipes. In my own life, I have eliminated foods made from processed white flour and have never looked back. With rare exception, I no longer indulge blindly in sweets, but still savor fresh seasonal fruits, especially the myriad berries and other fruits that are relatively low in carbohydrates.

Although complex carbohydrates are an integral part of the broad Mediterranean kitchen, food in this part of the world is by no means limited by its reliance on bread, pasta, rice, and other carb-rich raw ingredients. Indeed, once you start to take a closer look at the food traditions throughout the Mediterranean it is easy to see that there is so much there, from fresh fish, lamb, poultry, pork, and other meats, to an endless array of vegetables and greens, dairy products, regional charcuterie, and more, to satisfy Americans' growing appetite for good- and low-carb food solutions.

Olive oil is an integral part of the Mediterranean table, and in this book it is called for in almost every recipe. Without the delicious liquid gold of the Mediterranean, so many traditional vegetable and legume dishes would be unpalatable. Olive oil is a salve that not only makes food taste good but also is good for us. It has been proven to help prevent heart attacks and strokes and also helps metabolize sugar and insulin.

Cheese is also part of the culinary culture of the Mediterranean, and in the spirit of moderation it appears frequently, but in small quantities, in this book. I follow a reasonable approach to indulging in cheese: If I savor it one day, I may forego it the next, thereby keeping a sense of balance and temperance in the way I eat. But the use of cheese, just as the use of olive oil, has affected the fat counts in the recipes. I have tried to keep the carbohydrate counts at less than 15 grams and the fat counts at less than 20 grams. Almost all of it is from unsaturated, good fat—extra virgin olive oil. It is important, though, to look beyond one or two recipes when cooking from these pages—follow the golden rule of moderation. If you surpass your desired fat intake one day, eat lean the next.

This book began with my own personal need to rein in a little excess weight without going on a dieting extreme. As I began to experiment with recipes, it did not take long to realize that I was savoring a Mediterranean diet without "white" carbs, and that there was an endless array of both traditional and tradition-inspired dishes that fit perfectly well within the framework of good-carb eating.

Much of what I began cooking was also food that I had to get on the dinner table for my own family, dishes that I did not spend hours preparing, but that I more or less put together, like everyone else who "has" to cook, for a typical quick weekday meal. I never rely on prefab raw ingredients (such as chopped frozen vegetables, which have no taste), though, or processed foods. Because I wanted the dishes in here to represent the Mediterranean both in spirit and in practice, and because I have learned that speed is not the virtue most Americans pretend it to be, I always opt for real ingredients, organic when possible. There are some things I despise, such as low-fat cheese, which is blatantly absent in most of these pages. In its stead is the real stuff, just savored in that most Mediterranean of ways, with moderation. Desserts are also missing from these pages. It was a conscious decision to omit them, for several reasons: First, I am not a pastry specialist and don't much enjoy the finicky aspect of dessert making; second, I loath the idea of using sugar substitutes, which, to this purist's mind-set, are in the same league as low-fat potato chips. I enjoy fruit of all sorts, but on the dessert front I follow the path of abstention, indulging now and again, but generally holding still in the face of temptation.

My own favorite dishes span the Mediterranean, although my point of reference is mainly Greek. Most of the food in these pages has a seasonal bent. I love fresh green bean salads embellished with small chunks of meat or seafood and flavored with garlic, for example. Spinach is one of my favorite winter greens and in the spirit of good-carb cooking I use it in a variety of ways—on its own, fresh, in salads, or cooked into soups. Cauliflower and broccoli appear in numerous recipes because they are carb-friendly and extremely versatile.

I also love easy braised or stewed meats garnished with Mediterranean additions like capers and olives or lemon and herbs, or perked up with cumin, one of my favorite spices. Pork is a popular meat in the Mediterranean and one of the most versatile, both because it can be cooked in many different ways without the danger of drying out and because it is a good match for the whole spectrum of Mediterranean seasonings. It is also one of the most versatile raw ingredients, traditionally savored over half a year in the form of sausages, charcuterie, and more.

Lamb, the quintessential Mediterranean meat, is not something I generally cook every day, but perhaps that has more to do with my own cultural bias—for Greeks lamb is most often a festive or Sunday dish. In this book, lamb appears both in simple, everyday dishes and in more time-consuming, slower-cooked recipes that are suitable for special meals and holiday feasts.

In a nod to one of Americans' favorite meats, I have included a large array of chicken recipes, from stews and braises to whole roasted birds with Mediterranean flavors to sautéed breasts and more. Perhaps more than any other meat, chicken lends itself to quick preparations.

Fish and seafood are a fundamental part of the Mediterranean table, but also one of the most problematic because the Mediterranean itself is becoming more and more devoid of marine life and because the region's fish is not easy to find across the Atlantic. As a result, I have tailored the fish and seafood recipes to American tastes and needs. Shrimp and filleted fish, for example, play a major role.

The gamut of Mediterranean foods that can be tailored to carb-conscious cooking is vast. For so many Americans, the flavors, techniques, and raw ingredients of the Mediterranean have become second nature. Carb-friendly eating is not just a flash-in-the-pan trend, but a way of life well in the mainstream. It makes perfect sense to marry the two.

The Good-Carb Mediterranean Pantry

Bread One of the difficulties in writing this book was just how to deal with bread, to strike a balance between the needs of people watching their carbs and the sacred place bread holds on every table in the Mediterranean basin. I have not included bread recipes in these pages, but bread is not necessarily taboo. There is wisdom in the Mediterranean bread traditions of yore. In other words, look for breads that are made with whole grains and steer clear of anything containing processed white flour.

Carbohydrates are the new dietary villain. What fat was to the zeitgeist of the 1980s carbs are to the present. But blaming one entire food group for all the troubles resting languidly around our waistline is a blind approach to food. There are bad carbs and good carbs. The bad stuff is generally refined. These are the carbs that are stuffed into processed foods, packaged foods, commercially produced bakery items, crackers, chips, pasta, and white bread. Good carbs, on the other hand, are what have always been traditional in the Mediterranean. Unrefined, or complex carbohydrates, are found in natural, unprocessed foods, such as whole grains, unhulled or brown rice, legumes, and starchy vegetables. These foods are packed with everything good that we need: fiber, vitamins, and minerals. They take longer to digest, and therein lies the foundation of all low-carb and good-carb diets.

There are dozens of recipes in this book for stewed and braised dishes. These dishes are typical of the Mediterranean, and they call out for a piece of bread to dip into the pot juices. You can indulge in that with restraint, but when you do make sure you are dipping with a piece of whole grain, bran, oat, rye, or barley bread. Stone-ground whole wheat breads and pita bread can also be savored on occasion. Avoid all white breads and anything that says "fortified" on it.

Canned foods Canned fish, including tuna, sardines, and anchovies come in handy when preparing quick meals and snacks in the spirit of the Mediterranean. Good quality tuna is a mainstay for anyone watching his or her carbs. I like the Spanish brand Ortiz. The tuna belly is excellent and extremely tender, but pricey. Ortiz also sells very good quality albacore. Sardines are also a favorite fish throughout the Mediterranean, and they are practical for last-minute snacks or additions to salads, such as the classic Greek salad. Look for sardines packed in olive oil. Anchovies, another Mediterranean staple, should also be packed in olive oil.

Capers   Look for small capers in brine from the Mediterranean. My favorites are the small, irregularly shaped Greek capers. In Greek and Middle Eastern food shops you will also find caper leaves, which make a lovely addition to salads. If you want to reduce the saltiness of capers or of their leaves, blanch them a few times and rinse under cold water. The same holds true for olives.

Charcuterie   One of the saving graces for me when I first started watching my carb intake was the fact that I could eat all the prosciutto in the world, so long as I trimmed off the fat. The Mediterranean is charcuterie heaven, but unfortunately much of the traditional charcuterie, such as Italian pork sausages and chorizo, is extremely high in fat. While you can indulge in an occasional slice of bresaola and really good mortadella, it is better to go for leaner cured meat products, such as prosciutto trimmed of fat and Spanish ham, such as Serrano, also trimmed. Stay away from most sausages, either fresh or dried, although there are one or two recipes that call for chorizo in limited quantity. A strip or two of lean cured pork and a few fresh vegetables drizzled with a touch of olive oil is sometimes all you need to hold you over until dinner.

Cured Fish   Including smoked trout, herring, and the like betrays my bias as a Greek cook, since Greeks indulge in all manner of smoked and pickled fish. You can find delicious pickled octopus and mackerel, as well as smoked trout and smoked herring (the latter is a longstanding import and much-loved treat), in Greek and Middle Eastern shops all over the United States. These fish come ready to eat and make a good addition to buffet spreads. Drizzle them with a little extra-virgin olive oil and lemon juice and half a meal is on its way to completion.

Dairy   In a part of the world where shepherding is just about the oldest profession, it is hard to dismiss the mind-boggling array of cheeses that exist from one end of the Mediterranean to the other, and harder still to contemplate substituting them with fat-free versions. I just can't do it. I prefer to indulge with restraint and moderation in a wedge of Parmesan than to eat three slices of fat-free American cheese. That said, there is a fair amount of cheese in this book and the way to counter its hefty fat content is simply not to eat it every day. If you cook, say, a Portobello "Pizza" Margherita one day, stay away from the dairy drawer for a few days after that. In a few recipes, though, where the cheese content tips the fat scales, I call for low-fat versions.

Cheese, like the charcuterie of the Mediterranean, provides ample choices for all sorts of snacks and quick meals. A little cheese, a handful of salad greens, a drizzling of olive oil, and that's lunch for me on many occasions.

There isn't enough room here to catalog all the cheeses of the Mediterranean, but there are broad categories and some are more suitable to others on a carb-conscious regime. Feta, certain fresh goat's milk cheeses, certain blue cheeses such as Roquefort, and Parmesan and mozzarella are generally accepted on the South Beach model diet, albeit in limited quantities.

Fruits   Both the South Beach and Atkins diets allow certain fruits, especially after the first two weeks of the program. In the Mediterranean, fresh *and* dried fruits are savored regularly. It is best to eat fruit in season and grown as close to home as possible. Savor it after a meal, as is tradition throughout most of the Mediterranean, or for breakfast or a midday snack. The best fruits for carb-counters are apples, apricots, blueberries, grapefruits, grapes, kiwis, nectarines, oranges, peaches, pears, plums, raspberries, strawberries, and tangerines. Dried apricots and prunes are also allowed. Stay away from watermelon, sweet cherries, raisins, and dried figs and dates.

Grains   The few grains and grain products called for in this book include brown rice, wild rice, bulgur wheat, and a barley rusk, like a hard tack, which is a very traditional bread product in Greece. Grains, the basis of the Mediterranean Diet pyramid, are fundamental to the eating traditions in this part of the world. In general, as long as they are whole, it is okay to eat them regularly. I have included no pasta or couscous recipes in these pages, for several reasons. Couscous is absent mainly because in a half-cup portion, chock-full of 18 grams of carbs, I didn't feel that I could produce a recipe that would come anywhere close to the luscious couscous dishes traditional to North Africa. On the pasta front, although I have experimented with whole-wheat pasta and diabetic pasta,

I wasn't thrilled with the outcome. So I have left the use of those two very Mediterranean foods to your own discretion, to be accompanied by simple sauces or fresh vegetables. Bulgur is filling and a little bit goes a long way. Ditto on brown rice, which has a delicious nutty flavor and is called for in limited quantities in a few soup recipes.

Herbs and spices   These are an important element in every Mediterranean cuisine, especially when preparing low-carb meals. Anything that enhances the flavor of food without adding calories and carbs is welcome. In the Mediterranean the palette of flavorings is one of the factors that helps delineate one region's cuisine from another. There are differences in the way herbs and spices are used throughout the region. In Greece and Italy, for example, herbs are more prominent flavoring agents than spices. Greek cooks tend to use more dried herbs than fresh, with the exception of dill, parsley, and mint, whereas Italian cooks tend to savor more fresh herbs. Greeks generally do not cook with basil and sage, both popular in Italy, but make more use of oregano, marjoram, and thyme. Provençal cooks use herbs with abandon, and many are counted among the region's favorites. As for spices, Turkish cooks relish certain types of hot pepper, and cumin is the national spice of Morocco. Sweet, aromatic spices, such as cinnamon, cloves, and allspice play a role in the cooking of both Greece and North Africa.

Buy small amounts of fresh herbs and whole spices and chop, grind, or pulverize them just before using to ensure maximum taste. Once dried and ground, spices and herbs tend to lose some of their initial flavor.

Olive Oil   As I write this it is a sparkling November day in Athens, right around the start of the olive season. The sidewalk outside my house and all around the neighborhood is spotted with the small black splotches of trampled olives. As they fall off the tree in this urban clime, no one collects them; in the countryside, though, a whole other picture emerges. Whether one is in the coastal towns of Turkey, the dusty hillsides of North Africa, the lush grey-green groves of Kalamata, Crete, or Tuscany, or almost anywhere else in the Mediterranean, November is a month of concentrated frenzy. Depending on the weather and temperature, the olive harvest usually begins sometime around October or early November and can last through the end of January. It is the time that people in this part of the world obsess about the region's most important crop. No other foodstuff in the Mediterranean is as basic as the olive and its oil.

For Mediterranean cooks, olive oil is a constant; it is one of the raw ingredients that bridges the differences between the cuisines of all the countries and peoples in Southern Europe, the Near and Middle East, and North Africa. For American cooks, though, olive oil is often viewed as a gourmet product, something to be savored with great economy, to be used sparingly over only the freshest seasonal salads, over cooked vegetables, fish, and the like. In this book, as in many Mediterranean cookbooks, almost all the recipes call for olive oil. Greeks boast the highest per capita consumption of olive oil in the world, at nearly twenty-two quarts per person annually. As an American Greek I probably am a little more prodigious in my use of olive oil than other Americans, and as a result the fat content in some of the recipes might seem higher than expected. You can reduce the amount of olive oil in most cases to one or two tablespoons per recipe, but the truth is that all Mediterranean food relies on the region's liquid gold to make the wealth of vegetables dishes, pulses, legumes, and protein-based meals more tasty.

Fats are divided into two types: saturated and unsaturated. The former includes the gamut of animal-based fats such as butter, cream, and lard, but also margarine and tropical vegetable oils such as palm oil and coconut oil. Saturated oils are so called because of the chemical structure of the molecules, which are completely covered—saturated—with hydrogen atoms. Unsaturated fats are either polyunsaturated or monounsaturated. Monounsaturated fat helps to reduce the level of LDL (low-density lipoproteins), or "bad" cholesterol while maintaining the "good" HDL (high-density lipoproteins) cholesterol. In other words, good cholesterol actually helps remove bad cholesterol from the arteries and hinders its deposits. Olive oil is comprised of anywhere between 53 and 83 percent monounsaturated fat, depending on the variety of olive from which the oil was produced. It contains more monounsaturated fat than butter, margarine, and all other cooking oils.

Olive oil is most closely associated with its positive affects on heart disease;

when olive oil replaces saturated fats in the diet, it may help reduce the risk of cardiovascular disease, breast cancer, and prostate cancer. Olive oil might also help to increase bone density, and there is consistent evidence that a diet rich in olive oil leads to a longer life span.

Olive oil, like all fat, whether good or bad, contains 120 calories, or about 13 or 14 grams of fat, per tablespoon.

One of the questions I am frequently asked when I teach cooking classes in the United States is what kind of olive oil to buy. I inevitably answer extra virgin, and usually qualify that even further by recommending Greek oil because almost 90 percent of the oil produced in Greece is extra-virgin and in American markets it continues to be a very good buy. But the truth is the best olive oil is the one you like best at a price you can afford, and price is not always a reflection of quality as much as it is a reflection of marketing strategy and savvy. Many cooks in the United States keep more than one olive oil on hand, saving their favorite or best for dishes where it will shine most, such as over a fresh seasonal salad, and using their more prosaic oils for cooking, sautéing, and frying. That's a perfectly reasonable approach.

On American supermarket shelves the oils you are most likely to find are either Italian, Spanish, Greek, and, lately, Turkish. The best-known oils are Spanish and Italian. The best buys in terms of the quality-price ratio are Greek. I especially like the oils that come from Siteia, in eastern Crete, and from Kalamata, both recognized as designated appellations of origin, which, like wines with specific appellations, means that the oils are produced under the most stringent quality controls from region-specific olive varieties.

The flavor and quality of an olive oil depend on many factors: the variety of olives from which it is pressed, the age of the tree, the soil, climate, altitude, harvesting techniques, and handling, among other things, determine the final quality of olive oil. It is nearly impossible to quantify the distinctions between Spanish, Italian, Greek, Turkish, Provençal, Moroccan, and other olive oils because it is impossible to generalize. The flavor of olive oil varies from microclimate to microclimate within each producing country, and approximately 98 percent of the olive oil produced in the world is produced in the Mediterranean.

There are, however, various grades of olive oil defined by their acidity levels and ways to judge quality that leave the more subjective matters of particular tastes unattested. The lower the acidity, which is a measure of the amount of oleic acid per 100 grams of olive oil, the better the oil. But you can't actually taste the acidity in an oil unless it has gone rancid; acidity is measured in the laboratory. The general umbrella term "virgin" olive oil refers to unprocessed or unrefined oils, which means that once the olives have been harvested they have not undergone any other treatment other than washing, decantation, centrifugation, and filtration.

According to the International Olive Council, olive oils are delineated and graded as follows:

Extra Virgin Olive Oil   This is the best grade of olive oil. It is virgin, or unprocessed, and has an acidity level not exceeding 1 percent. Extra virgin olive oils must also have a perfect aroma, flavor, and color.

Virgin Olive Oil   This is also a virgin, or unprocessed olive oil, with an acidity level of not more than 2 percent and again with a perfect aroma, flavor, and color.

Olive Oil   This is a blend of refined and virgin olive oil. Oils marketed under the general grade "olive oil" must have an acidity level of not more than 1½ percent. The grade "olive oil" is oil in which flavor and aroma are less than perfect; it is refined so that it becomes a neutral product bland in every aspect—flavor, aroma, and color. This bland, refined oil has to be blended with virgin oil to make it more palatable.

Olive-Pomace Oil   This is not an olive oil and under no circumstances should it be labeled or presented as olive oil. It is refined oil that is extracted from the olive pomace—the pits and skins—that remains after pressing. This oil should have an acidity of not more than 1½ percent. Like ordinary olive oil, it is flavored with small quantities of virgin olive oil.

The range of tastes and flavors in olive oils is vast. There are various styles of olive oil, ranging from very sweet and mild to very bitter and pungent. Pepperiness is another flavor component, but it is often incorrectly assumed that good olive oil should be very peppery. There are excellent oils in all styles; choosing one is a matter of personal preference.

The quality of olive oil will be affected by the way in which the oil is stored. Excessive heat or humidity, as well as direct light, will adversely affect a bottle of olive oil. It is best to store olive oil in a cool, dark place where it will last, if properly taken care of, for up to two years.

Olives   This fruit is an integral part of the Mediterranean table and there are dozens of different varieties of table olives. Olives, like their oil, are beneficial to health. They are rich in monounsaturated acid—oleic acid—as well as vitamin E, which may reduce the risk of heart disease and some forms of cancer. Olives are also a good source of calcium, magnesium, and potassium. The only drawback in eating olives is their salt content, but extensive soaking or blanching allays their saltiness to a certain extent.

Olives also are rich in antioxidants; the amount varies depending on factors such as the variety of olive, the degree of ripeness at the time of harvest, and the soil in which they are grown. Increasing evidence points to the cancer-fighting properties of antioxidants and their positive effects in dealing with arteriosclerosis. Olive oil also contains antioxidants, but less than olives because some of their antioxidants are washed away during processing.

The olive is a drupe, like the peach and the plum. It is relatively low in sugar (2.6 to 6 percent) and high in oil content (12 to 30 percent). There are dozens of table olive varieties around the Mediterranean and several broad categories into which each fits. There are green olives, for example, such as the Spanish Manzanilla, the French Picholine, and the Greek cracked greens and Halkidiki olives. Green olives are harvested during a point in the ripening cycle at which they have reached full size but have not yet changed color. Each of these varieties and many more are processed slightly differently, an issue too complicated to detail here. Then there is a whole range of semi-ripe olives picked just at the point when the fruit is starting to change from green to black. Ripe olives are those that are harvested when the fruit is almost fully ripe. They include a whole range of black olives, such as the well known Kalamata olive. Finally, there are the wrinkled and thick-skinned olives, such as the Moroccan wrinkled olive and the Greek throumba, which are picked when they have ripened fully on the tree. These olives generally are not soaked in brine solutions as are all of the above, but layered directly in barrels with dry salt, which causes them to dehydrate partially and wrinkle even more.

Olives are consumed for the most part throughout the Mediterranean as a unique treat and snack, although their place in cooked dishes varies tremendously from country to country.

Nuts Some nuts are better than others for people watching their carbs. Chestnuts are almost an automatic no-no since they are extremely high in carbs (about 42 percent). Pine nuts contain about 12 percent carbohydrate; almonds about 20 percent; walnuts about 15 percent; and pistachios about 19 percent. In limited quantities nuts make for good snacks and add texture and flavor to all sorts of dishes, especially salads.

Sesame seeds These are one of the oldest and most traditional foods in the Mediterranean. They are a good low-carb addition to salads and other foods. Unhulled sesame seeds are made up of about 25 percent protein and about 4 percent fiber. They are high in fat—about 14 percent—but it is unsaturated fat. They are also an excellent source of calcium (about six times more than milk), iron, and vitamins B and B_6. Because of their high oil content, sesame seeds go rancid easily. It is best to store them in the refrigerator. Thanks to the popularity of Asian cuisine in America, sesame oil has become popular, too. Like olive oil it is an unsaturated fat, but it is not used readily in the Mediterranean and simply does not have the same complexity of flavors that extra virgin Mediterranean olive oil boasts.

Eggs for Breakfast, Brunch, and Dinner

A

S SURELY AS AMERICANS ARE APT TO HAVE A BREAKFAST of eggs and bacon or ham, Mediterraneans generally savored their eggs later on, as a light brunch or dinner. For low-carb acolytes the wealth and variety of egg dishes in the Mediterranean offer a treasure trove of acceptable and delicious recipes.

Eggs are important throughout the Mediterranean, and they have been since time immemorial. Starting in the easternmost reaches of the Mediterranean basin and ending on the Mediterranean shores of Spain and Morocco, eggs are cooked in countless different ways.

In Turkey, it was a simple but demanding egg dish that decided the fate of a palace cook. On the fifteenth day of Ramadan, the sultan traditionally left the palace to pay homage to a cloak that was thought to have been worn by the Prophet Mohammed. Upon his return, he ate a modest dish of eggs fried in a nest of spiced caramelized onions. If the dish was well prepared, the cook who made it would be appointed head of the royal pantry. Today, eggs cooked with onions are still a popular Turkish dish, as are poached eggs served with yogurt. To lower the carb content, you could substitute sour cream for yogurt. One of my favorite Turkish egg recipes is for Spicy Turkish Scrambled Eggs (page 24); it is similar to a Greek dish called strapatsatha.

Eggs are very popular throughout the Middle East and cooks approach them as a kind of culinary carte blanche. Hard-boiled eggs are embellished with all sorts of spices, especially cumin, coriander, and cinnamon and often sold as street food throughout the region. Whole eggs in the shell are often included in stews and other stovetop dishes, such as soups; they are added at the start so that as they simmer they can absorb all the flavors of the dish. Hard-boiled eggs are often used as a garnish for myriad stews and salads, again, all over the region but mostly in the Middle East and in Spain, as a result of the Moorish influence.

Omelets are a quick meal for people all over the Mediterranean, seldom made for breakfast but often prepared for lunch or for a light fast dinner. In most of the Mediterranean omelets are hearty, thick, and rather dry, as opposed to the fluffy, creamy omelets prepared by the French. In France omelets are eaten hot; in most of the rest of the Mediterranean they can be served either hot or at room temperature. In Greece, omelets go by various names and can include anything from sausage to spinach. They can be cooked in a skillet or baked; they are seldom folded but served whole, almost like a pan-fried pie. The omelet's closest relative, the frittata, is a dish that comes in many variations all over Italy. In Piedmont during truffle season, it might be served with a shaving of the region's famous white truffles; in Friuli, omelets are the midday workman's snack and are usually made into thick, hearty concoctions all crusty and brown on the surface and creamy within. One might find them fried in butter, lard, or goose fat. In the rest of Italy, olive oil is usually used to fry a savory frittata; in most other places outside Friuli, omelets are thin as crêpes.

Arguably the best-known egg dish in the whole Mediterranean is the Spanish tortilla, although eggs in all their guises are one of the most basic raw ingredients in all of Spanish cuisine. The classic tortilla Española contains the taboo (for low-carbers) potato, but there is no dearth of other tortilla dishes to sate the palate. Spanish egg dishes tend to be hearty and robust. Echoing a pan-Mediterranean custom, eggs are rarely eaten for breakfast but are considered more suitable as a midday snack or quick dinner. The Spanish, like the Greeks, adore their fried eggs, too, in olive oil, a treat one can find, like the tortilla, in most eating establishments all over Spain. Eggs make for an easy meze or tapa, usually in the form of an omelet, and often served in small wedges, perhaps with a few olives and a salad.

Eggs from the Skillet

Eggs on a Bed of Sautéed Mushrooms

Greek brunch is a filling affair. This is one of our Sunday family favorites.

2 servings

2 tablespoons extra virgin olive oil

½ cup sliced red onion

1 small garlic clove, minced

16 large button mushrooms, trimmed and cut into ⅛-inch slices

1 teaspoon dried thyme

½ teaspoon dried oregano

Salt and freshly ground black pepper

4 large eggs

⅓ cup finely crumbled feta cheese

Heat 1 tablespoon olive oil in an 8-inch nonstick skillet over high heat. Add the onions and garlic and sauté for 2 to 3 minutes, stirring frequently so they don't burn. Add the mushrooms, thyme, oregano, and salt and pepper to taste, and cook, stirring, until the mushrooms wilt a little but are still al dente, 4 to 5 minutes. Remove the mushrooms and divide evenly between 2 serving plates.

Wipe the skillet clean. Heat 1½ teaspoons olive oil. Break the eggs two at a time in the skillet as you would to make sunny-side-up eggs. Season lightly with salt and pepper. As soon as the white and yolk begins to set, flip the egg and sprinkle the whites with half the feta. Cover the skillet for a minute and cook until the feta is melted. Remove and place the egg on top of the mushrooms. Repeat with the remaining eggs and feta. Serve warm.

PER SERVING: Calories 441; Fat 33g (Saturated 10g); Cholesterol 547mg; Sodium 1,030mg; Carbohydrates 14g; Fiber 3g (Digestible Carbohydrates 11g); Protein 25g.

Scrambled Eggs with Garlic, Basil, and Gruyère

Scrambled eggs with a cheese that melts as well as Gruyère are an irresistible treat, for brunch, lunch, or dinner. Serve with a simple green salad or with one of the robust tomato or red pepper salads, or with a side dish of Horta *(page 92) or other cooked greens.*

2 servings

2 teaspoons olive oil

2 garlic cloves, smashed

4 large eggs

I tablespoons light cream

2 tablespoons finely chopped fresh basil

2 tablespoons grated Gruyère

Heat the oil in a large, heavy, preferably nonstick skillet over low heat. Add the garlic and cook until golden, but don't let it burn.

Beat together the eggs, cream, 2 tablespoons water, the basil, and cheese in a large bowl. Pour the egg mixture into the skillet over the garlic. Scramble lightly and cook until fluffy and soft but not runny. Divide between 2 plates and serve.

PER SERVING: Calories 237; Fat 18g (Saturated 6g); Cholesterol 437mg; Sodium 152mg; Carbohydrates 3g; Fiber 0g (Digestible Carbohydrates 3g); Protein 15g.

Sunnyside Up Eggs in Tomato Sauce
with Greek Fried Potato Skins

Okay, so the silver-dollar-shaped potatoes fried in olive oil are off limits to low carbers, but fried potato skins are an excellent alternative, offering a fraction of the carbs without skimping on the sinful flavor.

2 servings

3 ripe tomatoes, seeded and coarsely chopped

I small garlic clove, smashed

2 tablespoons fresh basil

I tablespoon extra virgin olive oil

Salt and freshly ground black pepper

3 large russet potatoes

4 large eggs

Olive oil for frying

Kosher salt

I scant teaspoon oregano

2 tablespoons grated kefalotyri or other hard yellow sheep's milk cheese

Place the tomatoes in a food processor and puree them, skins and all. Add the garlic, basil, 2 tablespoons extra virgin olive oil, salt and pepper to taste and pulse to combine. Place in a large skillet over low heat and cook, covered, for 20 to 25 minutes, or until the sauce is thick and pulpy.

Meanwhile, wash and scrub the potatoes very well and pat dry. Using a sharp potato peeler, peel off the skin in spirals. Place the skins in a bowl filled with ice water for 15 to 20 minutes. Drain and blot dry on paper towels. Save the potatoes for another use.

Fill another heavy skillet with olive oil to reach a ½ inch up the sides. Heat the oil over high heat to 375°F. To test, drop a small piece of the potato skin into the hot oil; if it sizzles, the oil is ready.

Carefully break the eggs into the tomato sauce. Cook over low heat until the eggs set in the sauce, about 7 to 8 minutes.

While the eggs cook, place the potato skins in the hot oil and fry them; it won't take more than a minute or so. Remove, drain the skins on paper towels, and place in a bowl. Sprinkle with kosher salt to taste, oregano, and grated cheese. Using a large spoon, carefully remove the eggs from the skillet and place on 2 serving plates. Divide the potato skins between the two plates and serve, with the sauce spooned on top.

PER SERVING: Calories 372; Fat 25g (Saturated 6g); Cholesterol 378mg; Sodium 1,376mg; Carbohydrates 22g; Fiber 4g (Digestible Carbohydrates 18g); Protein 16g.

Spicy Turkish Scrambled Eggs

This dish is often served with a dollop of thick yogurt sauce on the side, but you can substitute sour cream, either full-fat or low-fat.

4 servings

1 tablespoon extra virgin olive oil

1 red onion, finely chopped

1 medium green pepper, cored, seeded, and finely chopped

1 hot green chile, seeded and cut into thin strips

3 ripe tomatoes, peeled, seeded, and chopped

Salt and freshly ground black pepper

4 large eggs

Heat the olive oil in a large, heavy, preferably nonstick skillet over medium heat. Add the onion and cook until soft, 6 to 7 minutes. Add the pepper and chile and continue cooking until soft, another 4 to 5 minutes. Add in the tomatoes, and salt and pepper to taste and cook uncovered, over low heat for 10 minutes.

Add the eggs, stirring them into the mixture to distribute. Cover the skillet and cook until the eggs are set but still fluffy and tender, about 7 to 8 minutes. Divide between 4 plates and serve.

PER SERVING: Calories 317; Fat 18g (Saturated 4g); Cholesterol 425mg; Sodium 720mg; Carbohydrates 25g; Fiber 4g (Digestible Carbohydrates 21g); Protein 16g.

Asparagus, Basil, and Tomato Frittata

Asparagus and eggs are often paired throughout the Mediterranean.

4 servings

12 thin fresh asparagus stalks, trimmed

6 large eggs

Salt and freshly ground black pepper

$\frac{1}{3}$ cup grated Parmesan

1 tablespoon extra virgin olive oil

2 scallions, whites and tender greens, thinly sliced

1 garlic clove, minced

1 ripe plum tomato, seeded and diced

2 teaspoons chopped fresh basil, plus additional leaves, for garnish

Set an oven rack about 8 inches from the broiler and preheat the broiler.

Bring a large pot of salted water to a rolling boil and blanch the asparagus for 2 minutes. Drain and immediately immerse the stalks in a bowl of ice water to cool. Drain again. Cut the asparagus into 2-inch pieces.

Whisk the eggs together with salt and pepper to taste, and the Parmesan in a large bowl.

Heat the olive oil in a large ovenproof skillet, preferably cast-iron over high heat, add the scallions and garlic, and sauté for 1 minute. Add the asparagus and cook for 1 more minute, stirring gently. Add the tomatoes and basil and toss gently. Pour in the eggs and tilt the pan so that they spread all over the surface. Reduce the heat to low and cook the frittata until the bottom is set, 6 to 8 minutes. Place the frittata under the broiler, and broil until the top is golden 6 to 8 minutes. Cut into wedges and serve, either hot or at room temperature.

PER SERVING: Calories 198;Fat 13g (Saturated 4g); Cholesterol 324mg; Sodium 543mg; Carbohydrates 5g; Fiber 1g (Digestible Carbohydrates 4g); Protein 15g.

Ground Lamb and Eggplant Omelet

In the eastern reaches of the Mediterranean, ground lamb is a meat for all occasions, used to stuff vegetables, to top open-faced and sealed pastries, and, here, in this unusual Egyptian recipe, to embellish an otherwise simple egg dish.

6 servings

1 large eggplant (about ½ pound), cut into ½-inch cubes
Salt
1 tablespoon olive oil
½ cup chopped onion
½ pound ground lean lamb, preferably from the shoulder
2 garlic cloves, minced
2 tablespoons tomato paste diluted with 2 tablespoons water
Freshly ground black pepper
8 large eggs
½ cup finely chopped flat-leaf parsley
1 scant teaspoon ground cumin
1 teaspoon ground coriander

Salt the eggplant cubes in layers in a colander and set aside for 1 hour. Rinse well and pat dry.

Heat the olive oil in a large nonstick skillet over medium heat, add the onions, and sauté for 4 to 5 minutes, until they soften. Add the eggplant and continue sautéing until the eggplant is lightly browned and tender. Using a slotted spoon, remove the eggplant-onion mixture and set aside.

Add the lamb to the skillet and cook, still over medium heat, stirring, until browned. Add the garlic and tomato paste mixture and season with salt and pepper to taste. Lower the heat and cook for about 20 minutes, until the lamb is cooked through.

While the meat is cooking, beat the eggs, parsley, cumin, coriander, and salt and pepper to taste together in a large bowl. Drain off as much of the fat from the skillet as possible. Add the eggplant and onion mixture and toss. Pour in the eggs and tilt the pan to distribute the eggs evenly all over the skillet. Reduce the heat to low, cover, and cook until the eggs are set, 10 to 15 minutes. Remove from the heat, cut into 6 wedges, and serve.

PER SERVING: Calories 190; Fat 11g (Saturated 3g); Cholesterol 303mg; Sodium 386mg; Carbohydrates 6g; Fiber 2g (Digestible Carbohydrates 4g); Protein 15g.

Spanish-Style Tuna and Roasted Red Pepper Tortilla

Serve this easily prepared tortilla as a main lunch or dinner course.

2 servings

---

2 tablespoons extra virgin olive oil

½ cup coarsely chopped onion

I roasted sweet red pepper in brine, drained and coarsely chopped

2 ripe plum tomatoes, seeded and diced

I scant teaspoon dried tarragon

One 7-ounce can light tuna in brine, drained well and flaked

4 large eggs

Salt and freshly ground black pepper

Heat I tablespoon olive oil in a large nonstick skillet over medium heat. Add the onion and sauté until wilted, 2 to 3 minutes. Add the pepper, tomatoes, tarragon, and tuna and stir to combine. Reduce the heat to low and cook for 5 to 6 minutes, until the juices from the vegetables evaporate. Remove the skillet from the heat and set aside for about 5 minutes to cool slightly.

Whisk the eggs and salt and pepper to taste together in a large bowl. Add the tuna mixture to the eggs. Wipe the skillet clean.

Add the remaining tablespoon olive oil to the skillet, heat over high heat, and pour in the egg mixture. Lower the heat to medium and tilt the skillet so that the egg is evenly spread over the entire pan. As soon as the bottom is set and lightly browned, place a large plate over the skillet and, using an oven mitt to protect your hand from the heat, flip the tortilla over onto the plate. Slide it back into the skillet to cook on the other side for another 2 to 3 minutes. The tortilla should be moist, not dry. Do not overcook. Remove from the skillet and serve immediately.

PER SERVING: Calories 401; Fat 25g (Saturated 5g); Cholesterol 451mg; Sodium 1,016mg; Carbohydrates 9g; Fiber 2g (Digestible Carbohydrates 7g); Protein 35g.

Baked Omelet with Chorizo and Vegetables

Here's another hearty Spanish egg dish that can be served easily as a quick and filling main course.

4 servings

2 teaspoons olive oil

One 6-inch piece lightly cured chorizo or other garlicky fresh Mediterranean-style sausage, diced fine

1 large ripe tomato, seeded and diced

1 garlic clove, minced

2 tablespoons finely chopped flat-leaf parsley

Salt and freshly ground black pepper

3 large eggs

3 egg whites

2 tablespoons grated Parmesan

Preheat the oven to 375°F. In an 8- or 10-inch ovenproof, preferably cast-iron, skillet heat the olive oil over medium heat and brown the chorizo lightly. Add the tomato and garlic and cook until most of the juices have evaporated, about 8 minutes. Add the parsley and season lightly with salt and pepper.

Meanwhile, whisk the eggs and whites with salt and pepper to taste in a large bowl. Pour over the contents of the skillet, tilting the skillet so the eggs are distributed evenly. Once the eggs begin to set slightly, sprinkle the cheese on top and transfer to the oven. Bake for about 10 to 15 minutes, or until set, moist but not runny. Remove from the oven, cool slightly, and serve.

PER SERVING: Calories 224; Fat 16g (Saturated 6g); Cholesterol 183mg; Sodium 737mg; Carbohydrates 4g; Fiber 1g (Digestible Carbohydrates 3g); Protein 15g.

Crustless Quiche with Broccoli, Tarragon, and Two Cheeses

I like to serve this with Greek fried potato skins and some diced fresh tomato on the side.

8 servings

2 teaspoons extra virgin olive oil, plus I teaspoon for oiling the pan

6 scallions, finely chopped

2 cups chopped broccoli florets

6 large eggs

½ cup light cream

Salt and freshly ground black pepper

I scant teaspoon dried tarragon

½ cup soft mild goat cheese, such as Montrachet

½ cup grated Gruyère

Preheat the oven to 350°F. Oil a 9-inch round, 2-inch deep nonstick or Pyrex pie plate pan with I teaspoon olive oil.

Heat the olive oil in a large skillet over medium heat, add the scallions and sauté for 3 to 4 minutes, until softened. Add the broccoli florets and cook for about 7 minutes, until softened.

Whisk together the eggs, cream, salt and pepper to taste, and the tarragon in a large bowl. Stir in the cheeses and broccoli. Pour the mixture into the quiche pan and bake, uncovered, for 35 to 40 minutes, until golden and set. Serve hot or at room temperature.

PER SERVING: Calories 170; Fat 13g (Saturated 7g); Cholesterol 183mg; Sodium 135mg; Carbohydrates 3g; Fiber 1g (Digestible Carbohydrates 2g); Protein 11g.

Roasted Red Pepper and Feta Soufflé

My friend Aris Kefalogiannis once asked me to develop a recipe for one of the products his company sells abroad, a roasted red pepper and goat's cheese tapenade. I tried it in a soufflé and it was both pretty and flavorful. I have reworked the dish here so that it calls for ingredients prepared from scratch. If you can find his pepper-cheese spread, marketed under the Gaea name, use it in lieu of the feta and roasted red peppers below. It makes the dish even easier to whip together.

8 servings

2 tablespoons extra virgin olive oil

2 tablespoons flour

2 cups skim milk

3 tablespoons dry white wine

5 egg yolks, lightly beaten

3 roasted red peppers, pureed

½ cup crumbled feta cheese

½ cup grated Gruyère

Salt

2 teaspoons fresh chopped basil

2 teaspoons fresh chopped thyme

7 egg whites

Freshly ground black pepper to taste

Heat the oven to 450°F. Lightly butter a 2-quart soufflé dish.

In a medium saucepan over medium heat, heat the oil until it sizzles. Add the flour and stir until it turns golden blond. Pour in the milk and wine. Whisk the mixture continuously over medium heat until it begins to simmer and thickens, about 2 to 3 minutes. Remove from heat.

Whisking all the while, pour the beaten yolks into the hot milk in a slow steady stream until thick. Add the roasted red peppers, cheeses, salt, basil, and thyme to the mixture and mix well.

Using an electric mixer, beat the egg whites until stiff peaks form. Add half the meringue to the milk and pepper mixture, folding it in with a rubber spatula using quick, light hand movements. Fold in the remaining whipped egg whites the same way. Season with pepper. Pour the mixture into the prepared soufflé dish and place on a rack in the center of the oven. Reduce the oven temperature to 375°F and bake the soufflé for about 35 minutes, or until it puffs up.

Note: The soufflé may also be baked in individual soufflé cups. It will need less time to bake, around 20 to 25 minutes.

PER SERVING: Calories 165; Fat 11g (Saturated 4g); Cholesterol 150mg; Sodium 367mg; Carbohydrates 6g; Fiber 0g (Digestible Carbohydrates 6g); Protein 11g.

Spanakopita Soufflé

The wealth of savory pies that make for one of the Mediterranean's greatest treats is largely off limits to low-carbers. Soufflés, however, are a satisfying alternative. I have taken most of the ingredients used to make Greece's gastronomic gift to diners the world over and turned it into something easy and elegant—and low-carb. Try this with a colorful salad, such as one of the tomato or red pepper salads on pages 62, 63, and 64.

4 servings

¼ pound crumbled Greek feta

½ cup ricotta or fresh Greek anthotyro cheese

4 whole eggs, separated

3 tablespoons very finely chopped scallion

1 cup finely chopped fresh spinach

¼ cup finely chopped fresh dill

Salt and freshly ground black pepper to taste

Pinch of nutmeg

4 egg whites

Preheat the oven to 425°F. Lightly butter a 2-quart soufflé dish. Mash the cheeses together in the bowl of an electric mixer. Using the whisk attachment, add the 4 egg yolks and whip at high speed until smooth. Transfer to a large bowl and wash and wipe the mixer bowl.

Mix in the scallion, spinach, and dill. Season with salt and pepper to taste and the nutmeg.

Beat the 8 egg whites in the bowl of an electric mixer at high speed until stiff peaks form. Fold the whites into the spinach-cheese mixture and pour the mixture into the soufflé dish. Bake for 25 to 30 minutes, until the soufflé puffs up in the dish and acquires a light golden color. Remove from the oven and serve immediately.

PER SERVING: Calories 224; Fat 15g (Saturated 8g); Cholesterol 254mg; Sodium 758mg; Carbohydrates 4g; Fiber 0g (Digestible Carbohydrates 4g); Protein 18g.

Spinach-Graviera Quiche
Without a Crust

This is a rich dish, perfect for a festive brunch or dinner. Graviera, the cheese highlighted in this recipe, is similar to Gruyère. Substitute Gruyère or any mild, nutty, sweet cheese in its place.

6 servings

---

2 teaspoons extra virgin olive oil, plus I teaspoon for oiling the quiche pan

3 cups cooked spinach

5 scallions, whites and tender upper greens, finely chopped

4 large eggs

2 large egg whites

½ cup light cream

Salt and freshly ground black pepper

½ teaspoon ground nutmeg

½ teaspoon cayenne pepper

⅔ cup grated Greek graviera

Preheat the oven to 350°F. Oil a 10-inch round pie plate with 2 teaspoons olive oil.

Squeeze the cooked spinach dry between the palms of your hands and finely chop.

Heat the olive oil in a large skillet over medium heat, add the scallions, and sauté, for 3 to 4 minutes, until softened. Remove from the heat.

Whisk together the eggs and whites, cream, salt and pepper to taste, the nutmeg, and cayenne in a large bowl. Stir in the cheese, spinach, and scallions. Pour the mixture into the pan and bake, uncovered, for 35 to 40 minutes, until golden and set. Serve hot or at room temperature.

PER SERVING: Calories 178; Fat 12g (Saturated 6g); Cholesterol 166mg; Sodium 358mg; Carbohydrates 6g; Fiber 3g (Digestible Carbohydrates 3g); Protein 12g.

Peppers Stuffed with Eggs and Prosciutto

Vegetables stuffed with eggs and then baked is a playful dish found in both Greece and Italy. In Greece, tomatoes tend to be the vegetable of choice, usually filled with beaten eggs, herbs, and cheese. In this version, prosciutto and Asiago give the dish its flavors.

6 servings

4 large eggs

2 large whites

2 tablespoons club soda

A few drops of hot pepper sauce

½ cup grated Asiago or other mild yellow cheese

½ cup diced prosciutto or Spanish ham, trimmed of fat

1 tablespoon finely chopped fresh basil

1 teaspoon dried thyme

Salt and freshly ground black pepper

6 medium green bell peppers, halved lengthwise, cored, and seeded

Olive oil for greasing the pan

Preheat the oven to 350°F.

In a large bowl, whisk together the eggs and whites, club soda, and hot pepper sauce. Stir in the grated cheese, prosciutto, basil, and thyme. Season with salt and pepper to taste.

Place the peppers in a lightly oiled ovenproof dish large enough to fit them snuggly. Divide the egg mixture among the pepper halves, leaving about ¼ inch room at the top of each half. Pour a little water into the dish, enough to come about ⅛ inch up the sides of the peppers. Bake, uncovered, for about 50 minutes to 1 hour, until the peppers are tender and the eggs set. Remove, cool slightly, and serve.

PER SERVING: Calories 150; Fat 8g (Saturated 3g); Cholesterol 161mg; Sodium 575mg; Carbohydrates 9g; Fiber 2g (Digestible Carbohydrates 7g); Protein 12.

Eggs Florentine on Cretan Barley Rusks
with Grated Haloumi

This is a recipe inspired from the 2004 Olympics. A similar dish, created by Chef Costas Tsingas, who oversaw the dining facilities for the athletes, was offered on the breakfast buffet for the duration of the games.

4 servings

One 10-ounce package frozen chopped spinach, defrosted

1 tablespoon extra virgin olive oil

Salt and freshly ground black pepper

6 tablespoons light cream

Pinch of grated nutmeg

½ cup grated Haloumi cheese

4 large eggs

2 doughnut-shaped Greek barley rusks

Defrost the spinach according to the package directions. Heat the olive oil in a large nonstick skillet over medium heat. Add the spinach, season with salt and pepper to taste, and cook until all the liquid has evaporated. Add the cream, nutmeg, and cheese. Lower the heat.

Using the back of a wooden spoon, make 4 hollows in the spinach. Carefully break one egg into each of them. Cook over low heat until the eggs are set to desired doneness, but they should not be runny.

As the eggs cook, break each of the barley rusks into 2 halves. Dampen the rusks under the tap and let the water drip off. Divide the rusk halves among individual serving plates. When the eggs are done, carefully divide the mixture with a spatula and set the spinach mixture and 1 egg over each of the rusks. Serve immediately.

PER SERVING: Calories 386; Fat 19g (Saturated 8g); Cholesterol 242mg; Sodium 464mg; Carbohydrates 33g; Fiber 7g (Digestible Carbohydrates 26g); Protein 18g.

Greek Briam Baked with Eggs

Briam is one of the classics of the Greek vegetarian table, a dish made with thinly sliced zucchini, tomatoes, potatoes, and peppers. Here the potatoes are omitted. When all the vegetables are baked, crisp and golden, I pour eggs over them, and once set, I flip the pan so that the dish looks like a vegetable tarte Tatin. You will need an ovenproof skillet, preferably enamelware or cast iron.

6 servings

Salt

2 medium zucchini, sliced into ⅛-inch rounds

1 tablespoon extra virgin olive oil

1 large red onion, thinly sliced

3 garlic cloves, minced

3 large ripe tomatoes, thinly sliced

2 large green peppers, cored, seeded, and cut into thin rings

Freshly ground black pepper

1 scant teaspoon dried oregano

5 large eggs

4 tablespoons grated Greek kefalotyri or Parmesan

Preheat the oven to 400°F.

Salt the zucchini slices, layer them in a colander, and leave to drain for 1 hour. To expedite this process place a weight such as a can over the zucchini. Rinse the zucchini under cold water and blot dry with paper towels.

Heat the olive oil over medium heat in a large, nonstick ovenproof skillet, add the onion, and sauté for 6 to 7 minutes, until soft and lightly golden. Add the garlic and cook for another minute. Remove the onion and garlic to a small bowl and set aside.

Starting at the center of the skillet and fanning your way outward to the periphery of the pan, arrange the vegetables in overlapping rings, alternating between each slice, so there is a tight, spiral of sliced zucchini, sliced tomato, and pepper rings. Season lightly with salt and pepper. Toss the onions and garlic over the vegetables and sprinkle with the oregano. Bake, uncovered, for 50 minutes to 1 hour, until the vegetables, especially the zucchini, begin to wrinkle and brown lightly.

Beat the eggs with 3 tablespoons water and the cheese in a large bowl. Season lightly with salt and pepper and pour into the hot skillet over the vegetables. Wearing an oven mitt, tilt the pan so that the eggs cover the entire surface evenly. Slide the pan into the oven and bake for another 10 to 15 minutes, or until the eggs are firm and golden. Remove and cool slightly.

Cut into wedges and serve directly from the skillet.

PER SERVING: Calories 151; Fat 8g (Saturated 2g); Cholesterol 180mg; Sodium 514mg; Carbohydrates 13g; Fiber 3g (Digestible Carbohydrates 10g); Protein 9g.

Two Hard-Boiled Egg Dishes

Hamine Eggs

In Greece at Easter, traditional cooks slowly simmer their eggs together with the skins of red onions, which imparts a regal purple color to the shells after hours of gentle cooking. Both Arabs and Jews have a similar custom. What Sephardic Jews call huevos haminados, *Arabs know as* beid hamine, *eggs that have been very slowly simmered for up to six hours in a pot filled with water and either onion skins or used tea leaves or coffee grinds. The onions may be either of the yellow or red skin variety; the former imparts a copper color, the latter an intense purple hue. There are several ways to do this. Some recipes call for simmering the eggs in the oven; others for cooking over low heat on the stove. Either way, a little olive oil added to the pot will slow down the evaporation process during the hours–long cooking process.*

8 servings

8 large eggs, at room temperature
Papery skins from 4 large yellow or red onions
Vegetable oil

Place the eggs in a medium pot large enough to fit them in 1 layer without too much room to move around. Add water to cover the eggs by 4 inches and add the onion skins. Pour in enough oil to cover the surface of the water. Bring to a gentle simmer then lower the heat to the lowest possible setting. Simmer for 4 to 6 hours, replenishing the water as necessary.

Remove, and once the eggs are cool enough to handle, peel them and serve, sprinkled with a little salt, over a green salad or by themselves.

PER SERVING: Calories 78; Fat 5g (Saturated 2g); Cholesterol 212mg; Sodium 62mg; Carbohydrates 1g; Fiber 0g (Digestible carbohydrates 1g); Protein 6g.

Hard Boiled Eggs
Resimmered in Saffron Water

Saffron-boiled eggs are great alone with a drizzling of olive oil and a little pepper. They make for a light snack with a few tomatoes slices and also are an excellent garnish on almost all the spinach and other green salads in this book.

3 or 6 servings

½ teaspoon saffron threads

1 teaspoon salt

6 hard-boiled eggs, peeled

Place 4 cups water in a medium pot. Bring to a gentle simmer and add the saffron and salt. Stir to dissolve. Gently drop in the eggs. Simmer for about 1 hour, or until the eggs acquire a deep golden color. Remove, cool, and serve.

PER SERVING: Calories 78; Fat 5g (Saturated 2g); Cholesterol 212mg; Sodium 450mg; Carbohydrates 1g; Fiber 0g (Digestible Carbohydrates 1g); Protein 6g. based on 6 servings, 1 egg each.

Small Plates of the Mediterranean

ONE OF THE GREAT PLEASURES OF THE MEDITERRANEAN table is its innate sense of conviviality, manifested in the tradition of sharing small plates of savory foods. It is a tradition shared by everyone in every region, and those small plates go by several names: meze and mezze in the Eastern Mediterranean, antipasti in Italy, and tapas in Spain.

On traditional tables, bread and alcohol, whether it's arak, ouzo, wine, or something else, would almost always accompany these small plates. For acolytes of the low-carb lifestyle, bread and most of those beverages are either off limits or limited to an occasional indulgence, but the food remains a pleasure.

Dips and spreads and salsa-type dishes make up a large portion of the Mediterranean's small plates, and I have included a handful in the following chapter, culled from traditions that span the region. I recommend that they be savored with crudités or with some of the low-carb crackers and rusks. One of my favorites is the Wasa wafer, even though it doesn't hail from the Mediterranean.

Eggplant is arguably the most versatile vegetable in the Mediterranean. The Turks alone boast over a thousand dishes made with eggplant. Eggplant figures prominently in the cuisine of Greece, Italy, Spain, and North Africa. One of the most delicious ways to prepare it is smoked or grilled and then pureed, a dish that come in many guises and is known by several names, depending on whence it hails. Arabs and Israelis know it as baba ghanoush; Greeks call it melitzanosalata. Somewhere along the line it became known as eggplant "caviar" in the United States. That's what I call it here, too. Although not a rarity, it is a delicacy.

I have borrowed ideas in developing some of the following recipes, too. Traditional Niçoise tapenade is a very specific condiment, made with black olives, anchovies, and various other ingredients; the word has been coopted to mean almost any kind of robust dip or spread. The two tapenades in this chapter have been inspired by retail food products that surfaced over the last few years as the gourmet food market exploded in Greece.

The handful of recipes in this chapter are meant to convey a spirit of togetherness and sharing. Many dishes are suitable for entertaining, whether in the form of a dinner party or buffet.

Chunky Green Olive and
Lentil Tapenade in Endives

Olives are nutritious, carb-friendly, and quintessentially Mediterranean. I often serve this tangy dip with celery sticks or sometimes with Wasa or other low-carb crackers.

10 servings or about 2½ cups

1 tablespoon blanched almonds
2 garlic cloves, pressed
2½ cups green olives (preferably Greek), pitted, rinsed well, and drained
½ cup cooked green lentils, drained
Finely grated zest of 1 lemon (preferably organic)
¼ cup finely chopped dill
Salt and freshly ground white pepper
2 tablespoons extra virgin olive oil
2 Belgian endives, trimmed and broken into leaves (about 20 leaves)
Lemon zest cut into julienne for garnish
Small dill sprigs for garnish

Place the almonds and garlic in a food processor and pulse on and off until the almonds are finely chopped. Add the olives and pulse on and off a few times to chop coarsely. Add the cooked lentils and pulse on and off once or twice, just to break them up a little without mashing them completely.

Transfer the mixture to a serving bowl, add the lemon zest, dill, salt and pepper to taste, and olive oil and stir to combine well. Spoon a scant tablespoon of tapenade into each of the endive leaves. Garnish with lemon zest and dill and serve.

PER SERVING: Calories 133; Fat 12g (Saturated 0g); Cholesterol 0mg; Sodium 1,108mg; Carbohydrates 7g; Fiber 1g (Digestible Carbohydrates 6g); Protein 1g.

Eggplant Caviar with Roasted Garlic and Red and Green Peppers

The love affair between the Mediterranean and eggplant has been going on for centuries. It's no surprise that from Middle Eastern baba ghanoush to Greek melitzanosalata, there are dozens of recipes for roasted or smoked eggplant puree. This is a great starter, a lovely accompaniment to grilled meats and chicken, and it also goes nicely with grilled or sautéed fish and shellfish.

8 servings

1 head garlic

2 large eggplants

1 small green pepper

1 small red pepper

4 scallions, trimmed

3 tablespoons fresh lemon juice

4 tablespoons extra virgin olive oil

Salt and freshly ground black pepper

1 tablespoon chopped fresh mint

2 tablespoons finely chopped flat-leaf parsley

Preheat the oven to 375°F. Wrap the entire head of garlic in aluminum foil and place it on the bottom rack of the oven. Roast for about 1 hour, or until the garlic is soft when pierced. Remove, set aside to cool, and turn on the broiler.

Prepare the vegetables. Place the eggplants on a shallow baking tray and puncture all over with the tines of a fork. Place the peppers and scallions on the same tray. Broil until the vegetables are lightly charred, turning several times so that they cook all over. The peppers and scallions will need less cooking time than the eggplant.

Remove the scallions and set aside to cool slightly. Remove the peppers, place them in a bowl, and cover. When they are cool enough to handle, peel and seed, reserving as much of their juices as possible. Coarsely chop the scallions. Place the peppers and scallions in a food processor.

Remove the eggplant from the broiler and let it cool slightly. Cut in half lengthwise and, using a tablespoon, scoop out as much of the pulp as possible. Place in the food processor and immediately sprinkle with the lemon juice.

Squeeze the pulp from each garlic clove into the food processor. Pulse on and off, drizzling in the olive oil, until the eggplant mixture is a thick puree with chunky specks of red and green pepper clearly visible. Do not over process. Season with salt and pepper to taste and pulse to combine. Transfer to a serving bowl and mix in the mint and parsley. You can make this dish up to 2 hours ahead. Serve with fresh vegetables such as celery sticks and Belgian endive leaves.

PER SERVING: Calories 94; Fat 7g (Saturated 1g); Cholesterol 0mg; Sodium 150mg; Carbohydrates 8g; Fiber 3g (Digestible Carbohydrates 5g); Protein 1g.

Green Olive, Fennel, and Cilantro Tapenade on Cucumbers

Unlike the previous green olive tapenade, this dip is smooth, not coarse. The trio of flavors is fragrant and the cucumbers add a neutral but cool backdrop to this simple dip.

8 servings

I tablespoon extra virgin olive oil

I small fennel bulb, finely chopped

I garlic clove, minced

3 cups green olives (preferably Greek), pitted, rinsed, and drained

1/4 teaspoon cayenne pepper

1/2 teaspoon freshly ground black pepper

2 tablespoons finely chopped fresh cilantro, plus whole leaves for garnish (optional)

2 teaspoons fennel seeds, ground

I tablespoon finely chopped orange zest

I to 2 cucumbers, peeled and cut into 1/2-inch rounds

Heat the olive oil in a small skillet over medium heat. Add the fennel and garlic and sauté until softened slightly, about 4 minutes. Remove and set aside to cool.

Place the olives in a food processor with the cooked fennel, cayenne, black pepper, cilantro, fennel seeds, and orange zest. Pulse on and off until the mixture becomes the consistency of a dense, chunky paste.

Place a scant teaspoon of the tapenade on the cucumber rounds, garnish with cilantro leaves if desired, and serve.

PER SERVING: Calories 127; Fat 12g (Saturated 0g); Cholesterol 0mg; Sodium 1,191mg; Carbohydrates 7g; Fiber 1g (Digestible Carbohydrates 6g); Protein 0g.

Roasted Pepper and Goat Cheese Spread

Again, all over the European end of Mediterranean, in one form or another, roasted red peppers are considered a natural partner to soft tangy cheese, such as chèvre. Feta works well here, too.

12 servings

6 large red peppers, roasted, peeled, seeded, and coarsely chopped, or 6 roasted red peppers in olive oil, drained and chopped

1½ cups fresh goat cheese, such as Montrachet

2 tablespoons extra virgin olive oil

2 teaspoons fresh lemon juice

Salt and freshly ground black pepper

Combine all the ingredients in a food processor and pulse on and off until the mixture becomes a dense, velvety spread.

Transfer to a serving bowl and refrigerate for 1 hour or up to 2 days. Serve with fresh vegetables such as cauliflower florets, Belgian endive leaves, or celery sticks.

PER SERVING: Calories 118; Fat 8g (Saturated 5g); Cholesterol 13mg; Sodium 203mg; Carbohydrates 6g; Fiber 2g (Digestible Carbohydrates 4g); Protein 6g.

Roasted Red Pepper Hummus

The idea for this dish came from a Middle Eastern deli on Manhattan's East Side.

8 servings

4 large red bell peppers, roasted, peeled, and seeded or 6 roasted red peppers
   in olive oil, drained and chopped
1 cup canned chickpeas, rinsed and drained
3 garlic cloves, minced
2 tablespoons tahini
2 tablespoons extra virgin olive oil
2 to 3 tablespoons fresh lemon juice
Salt
½ teaspoon cayenne pepper, or more to taste

Place the red peppers, chickpeas, garlic, tahini, olive oil, and lemon juice in a food processor and process until smooth. Season to taste with salt and cayenne.

Transfer to a bowl and serve with a selection of raw vegetables such as celery, Belgian endive leaves, and cauliflower florets.

PER SERVING: Calories 105; Fat 6g (Saturated 1g); Cholesterol 0mg; Sodium 206mg; Carbohydrates 11g; Fiber 3g (Digestible Carbohydrates 8g); Protein 3g.

Small Vegetable Plates

Caponata

This Italian classic goes well with all sorts of dishes, but I often savor it with grilled meats and poultry.

4 servings

1 large eggplant (about 1½ pounds), cut into ½-inch cubes

Salt

3 tablespoons extra virgin olive oil, plus more for drizzling (optional)

1 medium red onion, coarsely chopped

2 garlic cloves, minced

2 large, ripe tomatoes, peeled, seeded, and cut into 1-inch cubes

1 tablespoon capers

2 tablespoons fresh julienned basil or chopped fresh oregano

Freshly ground black pepper

1 tablespoon balsamic vinegar

2 tablespoons chopped flat-leaf parsley, for garnish

Season the eggplant cubes generously with salt and place in a colander. Place a plate or other weight on top and set aside to drain in the sink for 1 hour. Rinse the eggplant and wipe dry with paper towels.

Heat 1½ tablespoons olive oil in a large nonstick skillet over high heat, add the eggplant, and brown lightly. Remove the eggplant from the skillet and set aside. Add the remaining 1½ tablespoons olive oil, reduce the heat to low, add the onions, and cook until lightly golden, about 15 minutes. Add the garlic and cook, stirring, for 1 to 2 more minutes. Stir in the tomatoes and return the eggplant to the skillet. Add the capers and basil. Season with salt and pepper to taste. Simmer gently for about 5 minutes, stirring occasionally with a wooden spoon. Stir in the vinegar and remove from the heat. Let cool slightly and serve, either warm or at room temperature, garnished with chopped parsley and a little olive oil, if desired.

PER SERVING: Calories 175; Fat 11g (Saturated 2g); Cholesterol 0mg; Sodium 458mg; Carbohydrates 18g; Fiber 6g (Digestible Carbohydrates 12g); Protein 3g.

Italian-Style Dry Roasted Cauliflower

Cauliflower is one of the salvation vegetables of low-carb eating. Yet like most people, I grew up believing that cauliflower is a vegetable destined only for blanching and boiling, and rarely for the oven. But the opposite is true. The dry heat of the oven inparts a nuttiness to this otherwise bland vegetable.

This simple recipe requires nothing at all beyond cutting the cauliflower into florets, tossing them with a little olive oil and coarse salt, and roasting in a medium-hot oven for a little less than an hour. The result is a side dish or starter that is excellent with most fish recipes and many of the aromatic lamb recipes in this book.

6 servings

---

1 medium cauliflower (about 2 pounds), cut into small florets

⅓ cup extra virgin olive oil

½ teaspoon cayenne pepper

Sea salt and freshly ground black pepper

2 to 3 tablespoons fresh lemon juice

Preheat the oven to 350°F.

Toss the cauliflower with the oil, cayenne, and salt and pepper to taste in a large bowl. Place in a shallow pan and bake, covered, for 45 minutes. Remove the cover and continue baking another 10 to 15 minutes, until lightly browned. Remove and serve hot or at room temperature, drizzled with lemon juice.

PER SERVING: Calories 130; Fat 12g (Saturated 2g); Cholesterol 0mg; Sodium 222mg; Carbohydrates 5g; Fiber 2g (Digestible Carbohydrates 3g); Protein 2g.

Roasted Eggplant Slices
with Anchovy Sauce

This classic Italian antipasto is best at room temperature. Leave it out for an hour or two, covered, before serving.

6 servings

1 large eggplant (about 1½ pounds), cut into ¼-inch slices
Salt
⅓ cup plus 1 tablespoon extra virgin olive oil
2 garlic cloves, minced
6 anchovy fillets
1 cup drained chopped plum tomatoes
2 tablespoons finely chopped flat-leaf parsley
2 tablespoons finely chopped fresh basil
2 tablespoons red wine vinegar, or more to taste

Layer the eggplant rounds in a large colander, salting each layer. Place a plate and a weight on top of the eggplant and set aside to drain in the sink for 1 hour. Remove the eggplant, rinse lightly, and pat dry with paper towels.

Preheat the oven to 450°F. Oil a large sheet pan and place the eggplant slices in a single layer in the pan. Brush with olive oil. Bake for 8 to 10 minutes on each side, or until golden and tender, taking care not to burn the eggplant.

While the eggplant is baking, prepare the sauce by heating 1 tablespoon olive oil in a medium skillet over medium heat. Add the garlic and sauté, stirring for about 1 minute, until it releases its aroma. Do not brown. Add the anchovies and mash them in the skillet with a fork. Add the tomatoes, raise the heat a little, and bring to a boil. Cover, reduce the heat to low, and simmer for 10 to 12 minutes, until the sauce is thick. Add the parsley, basil, and vinegar. Cook, uncovered, for 2 minutes, stirring, then remove from the heat.

Remove the eggplant slices from the oven and arrange about half, or as many of the slices as will fit in 1 overlapping layer, on a large plate. Spoon half the sauce over them and top with remaining eggplant and then the remaining sauce.

PER SERVING: Calories 260; Fat 19g (Saturated 3g); Cholesterol 38mg; Sodium 1,979mg; Carbohydrates 9g; Fiber 3g (Digestible Carbohydrates 6g); Protein 14g.

Spanish-Style Mushrooms with Bacon, Garlic, and Wine

This dish and the following one are simple recipes for quickly cooked savory mushrooms.

6 side-dish servings

⅓ cup diced lean bacon

2 garlic cloves, minced

1 pound small button mushrooms, trimmed

½ cup dry white wine

Salt and freshly ground black pepper

Pinch of cayenne pepper

¼ cup finely chopped flat-leaf parsley

Place the bacon in a large, deep skillet over medium heat and cook until it begins to brown. Add the garlic and cook until the garlic is glossy and soft, about 2 minutes. Add the mushrooms and toss to coat with the bacon fat. Pour in the wine. As soon as the wine steams up, season with salt and pepper to taste and the cayenne.

Cover the skillet, raise the heat to high, and cook until most of the pan juices evaporate and the mushrooms are tender. Toss in the parsley, stir, and remove from the heat. Serve either warm or at room temperature.

PER SERVING: Calories 38; Fat 2g (Saturated 1g); Cholesterol 2mg; Sodium 242mg; Carbohydrates 4g; Fiber 1g (Digestible Carbohydrates 3g); Protein 3g.

Spicy Spanish Mushrooms with Chilies and Garlic

6 side-dish servings

1 tablespoon extra virgin olive oil

3 large garlic cloves, slivered

1 small dried chile (with seeds), chopped

1 pound small button mushrooms, trimmed

Salt

½ cup beef or chicken broth

1 tablespoon fresh lemon juice

¼ cup finely chopped flat-leaf parsley

Heat the olive oil in a large, deep skillet over low heat. Add the garlic and chile and cook until the garlic begins to turn a light gold, about 3 minutes. Add the mushrooms, toss to coat in the oil, and season with salt to taste. Raise the heat and pour in the broth. Cover partially and cook for about 8 minutes, until the mushrooms are tender.

Stir in the lemon juice and parsley and continue cooking another 2 to 3 minutes, until the parsley wilts. Serve hot or warm with all the pan juices.

PER SERVING: Calories 44; Fat 3g (Saturated 0g); Cholesterol 0mg; Sodium 236mg; Carbohydrates 4g; Fiber 1g (Digestible Carbohydrates 3g); Protein 3g.

The Mediterranean Garden in a Bowl

T WO THINGS MAKE THE QUALITY OF SALADS ALL OVER THE
Mediterranean unsurpassable: the quality and variety of
seasonal, regional vegetables and the quality and profuse-
ness of olive oil.

From Istanbul to Madrid, in cities and countryside alike, one of
the great pleasures of life in this part of the world, and something
all cultures share, are the markets. The vegetables and fruit markets
that anchor major cities or that travel from neighborhood to neighborhood offer the best glimpse in the world of the Mediterranean's
love affair with all things fresh, seasonal, and of the earth.

There isn't a country in the Mediterranean that doesn't boast a
great summer tomato salad. Winter salads from places as far afield
as Italy and Turkey rely on vegetables that are served either raw or
boiled. The salad bowl changes with the seasons, so summer is a bo-
nanza of tomato, pepper, and cucumber salads, which gives way to

more autumnal greens salads, wintry cabbage salads, and, finally, delicate spring salads that call for new spring vegetables, such as tender lettuces, young fresh herbs, and asparagus.

Although in every culture in the Mediterranean seasonality is revered as a cornerstone not only for the salad bowl but also for proper cookery at large, the place of the salad on the table changes from country to country. In Greece, the Middle East, and North Africa, salad is not served as a separate course so much as part of a spread including other dishes, all present at the same time on the table, often at the beginning of the meal. The colors and textures of salads in these parts of the world are vibrant and varied. The role of the salad is meant to whet the appetite for further eating rather than cleanse the palate or expedite digestion. By contrast, in Spain salad is almost always served as a first course, whereas in Italy and France it usually is considered a precursor to the meal's impending end, and served after the main, or second, course. It is meant to relax and cool down the palate.

A salad in the Mediterranean is also open to wide interpretation. It can be made of almost anything, from fresh raw or boiled vegetables to meat and seafood, legumes, and bulgur wheat. It is usually simple, often filling and down to earth. Dressings are generally a simple duet of extra virgin olive oil and lemon juice or vinegar. The olive oil should be of excellent quality, extra virgin, cold pressed.

I have tried to give a sense of the breadth of salads from one of the world's most fecund gardens. Always use the freshest, seasonal ingredients for your salad. Try to buy local ingredients, and have at least one great olive oil on hand when dressing them.

Summer Salads

Garden Salad with Sardine Fillets

This is essentially a spruced up Greek horiatiki, *or typical "villager's" salad.*

6 servings

1 hothouse cucumber, unpeeled, quartered lengthwise and diced

4 large tomatoes, seeded and diced

1 small red onion, finely chopped

½ cup chopped flat-leaf parsley

1 bunch arugula, stems trimmed and leaves chopped

4 sardine fillets packed in olive oil, drained and chopped

4 whole sardine fillets packed in oil, drained

The dressing

¼ cup extra virgin olive oil

1 tablespoon fresh lemon juice

Salt and freshly ground black pepper

Combine all the vegetables, herbs, and chopped sardines in a serving bowl. Toss to combine. Place the 4 whole sardines fillets decoratively on top of the salad.

To make the dressing, whisk together the olive oil, lemon juice, and salt and pepper to taste. Pour the dressing over the salad and serve.

PER SERVING: Calories 150; Fat 11g (Saturated 2g); Cholesterol 23mg; Sodium 290mg; Carbohydrates 8g; Fiber 2g (Digestible Carbohydrates 4g); Protein 6g.

Andalusian Tomato Salad

Salads don't get much simpler than this. It's best to use locally grown organic vegetables for this, and all the fresh salads in this chapter. What's at work in this recipe is a medley of different ingredients that make this simple dish an exercise in opposites: sweet tomatoes, onions, and peppers are countered by briny green olives, garlic, and vinegar.

6 servings

4 large ripe tomatoes, cut into 6 wedges each

I Spanish onion, sliced into thin rings

2 red bell peppers, cored, seeded, and cut into thin rings

⅓ cup good-quality green olives, pitted if desired

The Dressing

¼ cup extra virgin olive oil

2 tablespoons sherry vinegar

I garlic clove, minced

Salt and freshly ground black pepper

¼ cup finely chopped flat-leaf parsley

Layer the salad in a serving bowl as follows: first the tomatoes, then the onion, followed by the peppers, and then the olives.

Whisk together the olive oil, vinegar, garlic, and salt and pepper to taste. Pour the dressing over the salad, let stand for 10 minutes at room temperature, sprinkle with the parsley, and serve.

PER SERVING: Calories 146; Fat 12g (Saturated 1g); Cholesterol 0mg; Sodium 428mg; Carbohydrates 12g; Fiber 3g (Digestible Carbohydrates 9g); Protein 2g.

Moroccan Spiced Tomato and Chile Salad

In Greece we have the ubiquitous Greek villager's salad; here is a distant cousin, from Morocco, which comes minus the Kalamata olives but with no dearth of bold flavored ingredients, including chiles.

6 servings

2 large green bell peppers

1 green or red chile

4 large ripe tomatoes, peeled, seeded, and diced

1 hothouse cucumber, peeled, seeded, and diced

1/3 cup chopped flat-leaf parsley

1/2 teaspoon ground cumin

2 tablespoons extra virgin olive oil

3 tablespoons fresh lemon juice

Salt and freshly ground black pepper

Light the broiler or grill and roast the peppers and chile, turning, until charred all over. Remove and place in a plastic bag. Once the peppers have cooled (wear latex gloves for the chile), peel off the skins, slit, and remove the seeds and stems. Coarsely chop the peppers and chile.

Combine the peppers, chile, tomatoes, cucumber, parsley, cumin, olive oil, lemon juice, and salt and pepper to taste in a serving bowl. Toss gently. Let stand for 15 minutes before serving.

PER SERVING: Calories 91; Fat 5g (Saturated 1g); Cholesterol 0mg; Sodium 209mg; Carbohydrates 12g; Fiber 3g (Digestible Carbohydrates 9g); Protein 2g.

Provençal Roasted Yellow Pepper
and Tomato Salad

This is a gorgeous, colorful paean to the Mediterranean table in summer.

6 servings

3 large yellow peppers
1 small bunch fresh basil, leaves only
2 garlic cloves, minced
Sea salt and freshly ground black pepper
¼ cup extra virgin olive oil
4 large ripe tomatoes, seeded and diced

Light the broiler or grill and roast the peppers, turning, until charred on all sides. Remove and place in a plastic bag for 5 minutes.

Remove the peppers from the bag, reserving their juices. Carefully peel the peppers. Cut in half lengthwise and then cut each half horizontally into 1-inch strips.

Place the basil, garlic, salt and pepper to taste, olive oil, and any juices from the peppers, strained, in a food processor and pulse on and off to make a smooth, thick dressing. Combine the peppers and tomatoes in a serving bowl, add the dressing, and toss gently to combine. Cover and let stand at room temperature for 30 minutes to 1 hour before serving.

PER SERVING: Calories 134; Fat 10g (Saturated 1g); Cholesterol 0mg; Sodium 205mg; Carbohydrates 12g; Fiber 3g (Digestible Carbohydrates 9g); Protein 2g.

Zucchini Carpaccio with Herbs and Sheep's Milk Cheese

In the summer, when we grow our own organic zucchini, we live off this salad. The zucchini is sliced into paper-thin shavings on a mandolin. It's light, robust, and filling.

6 servings

2 medium zucchini

¼ cup extra virgin olive oil

3 tablespoons fresh strained lemon juice, or more to taste

I teaspoon finely chopped fresh oregano

Sea salt and freshly ground black pepper

6-ounce piece of Parmesan or Cretan graviera

Scrub the outside of the zucchini under cold running water and trim off the ends. Using a mandolin or food processor, slice the zucchini lengthwise into paper-thin pieces.

Whisk together the olive oil, lemon juice, oregano, and salt and pepper to taste in a medium bowl.

Arrange the zucchini in overlapping slices on a large platter. Drizzle with the dressing. Let stand for 30 minutes to I hour to marinate.

Using a vegetable peeler, shave the Parmesan into thin strips and strew them decoratively over the zucchini. Serve immediately.

PER SERVING: Calories 202; Fat 16g (Saturated 6g); Cholesterol 19mg; Sodium 648mg; Carbohydrates 4g; Fiber Ig (Digestible Carbohydrates 3g); Protein 11g.

Green Bean Salad with Onions and Ham

Use young, tender greens for this salad, and trim them well.

6 servings

1 pound green beans, trimmed

¼ cup extra virgin olive oil

3 tablespoons red wine vinegar

Salt and freshly ground black pepper

1 large white onion, minced

2 roasted red peppers in brine, drained and diced

2 ounces Spanish ham or prosciutto di Parma, chopped

1 hard-boiled egg, finely chopped

⅓ cup chopped flat-leaf parsley

Steam the green beans for about 8 minutes, until tender but al dente, or blanch them in salted water (it helps retain their color) for 6 to 7 minutes. Drain in a colander and rinse with cold running water. Pat dry.

In a small bowl, whisk together the olive oil, vinegar, and salt and pepper to taste.

Place the green beans in a serving bowl. Top with the minced onion, peppers, ham, egg, and parsley. Pour the dressing over the salad, toss, and serve.

PER SERVING: Calories 152; Fat 11g (Saturated 2g); Cholesterol 44mg; Sodium 401mg; Carbohydrates 9g; Fiber 3g (Digestible Carbohydrates 6g); Protein 5g.

Green Bean, Mushroom, and Smoked Ham Salad

Another salad, culled from the vast repertory of Italian antipasti and salads, which could easily hold its own as a main course.

8 servings

1 pound young, tender fresh green beans, trimmed

⅓ cup extra virgin olive oil

2 tablespoons sherry or good-quality red wine vinegar

Salt and freshly ground black pepper

1 garlic clove, minced

¼ pound medium button mushrooms, sliced

3 ounces lean smoked ham, diced

1 large ripe tomato, seeded and diced

½ cup fresh basil cut into thin ribbons

Bring a large pot of salted water to a rolling boil and blanch the green beans for about 4 minutes, until tender but al dente. Drain and rinse under cold water in a colander. Pat dry.

In a small bowl, whisk together the olive oil, vinegar, and salt and pepper to taste.

Combine the beans with the garlic, mushrooms, ham, diced tomato, and basil. Pour the dressing over the salad, toss gently, and serve.

PER SERVING: Calories 123; Fat 10g (Saturated 1g); Cholesterol 6mg; Sodium 384mg; Carbohydrates 7g; Fiber 2g (Digestible Carbohydrates 5g); Protein 4g.

Winter Salads

Spiced Raw Carrot Salad

Serve this salad with pungent, robust accompaniments, such as a wedge of feta cheese, or with mild-flavored dishes such as grilled or roasted chicken.

8 servings

8 large carrots,
1 small garlic clove, minced
4 tablespoons ground walnuts
½ teaspoon ground cinnamon
½ teaspoon ground cumin
¼ teaspoon cayenne pepper, or more to taste
⅓ cup extra virgin olive oil
Juice of 1 lemon
Salt
¼ cup shredded fresh mint

Shred the carrots.

Combine the carrots, garlic, walnuts, cinnamon, cumin, cayenne, olive oil, lemon juice, and salt to taste in a serving bowl. Cover and let stand for 1 hour at room temperature or in the refrigerator for up to 8 hours. Just before serving, toss in the mint and serve.

PER SERVING: Calories 130; Fat 11g (Saturated 1g); Cholesterol 0mg; Sodium 172mg; Carbohydrates 9g; Fiber 3g (Digestible Carbohydrates 6g); Protein 1g.

Spinach Salad with Hard-Boiled Eggs, Cumin, and Garlic

Raw spinach salads are one my personal favorites. I always recommend organic spinach because spinach happens to be one of the vegetables that pesticides cling to easily. Even repeated washing won't dispel them.

6 servings

---

2 ripe tomatoes, peeled, seeded, and cut into ¼-inch cubes

½ teaspoon ground cumin

1 small garlic clove, minced

Pinch of cayenne pepper

½ teaspoon sweet Hungarian paprika

⅓ cup extra virgin olive oil

2 tablespoons sherry vinegar

½ pound spinach or escarole, coarsely chopped

Salt and freshly ground black pepper

3 hard-boiled eggs, quartered

12 salt-cured Moroccan or Thassos olives

Combine the tomatoes, cumin, garlic, cayenne, paprika, half the olive oil, and the vinegar in a small bowl and allow to marinate for 30 minutes.

In a salad bowl, toss the greens with the remaining olive oil and salt and pepper to taste. Season the tomato mixture lightly with salt and pepper. Toss with the greens.

Place the eggs and olives decoratively over the top of the salad and serve.

PER SERVING: Calories 186; Fat 17g (Saturated 3g); Cholesterol 106mg; Sodium 382mg; Carbohydrates 5g; Fiber 2g (Digestible Carbohydrates 3g); Protein 5g.

Spanish Beet and Onion Salad

Beets are one of the quintessential Mediterranean vegetables—earthy, hardy, and really good for you. In this dish, a classic on the Spanish table, the sweetness of the beets is nicely balanced by the pungency of the raw onions and by the acidity in the dressing. Because of their innate sweetness and thus relatively high carb count, beets may not be a vegetable low carbers indulge in often, but this dish adheres to one of the golden rules of the Mediterranean: nothing in excess. The counts are fine, and a little indulgence now and again makes us all feel good.

6 servings

---

4 medium beets

Salt and freshly ground white pepper

Very finely grated orange zest from half of a medium orange

½ large red onion, thinly sliced

3 tablespoons extra virgin olive oil

2 teaspoons sherry vinegar

1 tablespoon chopped fresh mint, for garnish

Cut away and discard the stem and root ends of the beets. Wash and scrub very well. Place the beets in a medium saucepan with ample salted water over high heat. Bring to a boil, reduce the heat, and simmer for 50 minutes to 1 hour, until tender. Remove, drain in a colander, and rinse under cold water. Peel the beets when they are cool enough to handle.

Using a sharp knife, cut the beets into very thin rounds.

Place about a quarter of the beets in a shallow serving bowl. Season with salt and pepper to taste and sprinkle lightly with the orange zest. Strew about a quarter of the onion slices over the top. Drizzle with 1 tablespoon olive oil and ½ teaspoon vinegar.

Repeat with the remaining onions, olive oil, and vinegar, finishing with a layer of onion slices. Garnish with the mint and serve.

Note: You can also layer the salad as indicated above without dressing or garnishing it. Cover with plastic wrap and refrigerate for 1 hour. The flavors of the beets and onions will marry better that way. Dress and garnish just before serving.

PER SERVING: Calories 80; Fat 7g (Saturated 1g); Cholesterol 0mg; Sodium 289mg; Carbohydrates 5g; Fiber 1g (Digestible Carbohydrates 4g); Protein 1g.

Spinach Salad with Ricotta Salata, Olives, Pine Nuts, and Tomatoes

Salads that couple fresh spinach with cheeses abound inside and outside the Mediterranean. In this salad, you can substitute the mild, buttery Greek manouri cheese or ricotta salata with something more robust, such as feta, Gorgonzola, or even Roquefort.

8 servings

2 tablespoons pine nuts

6 cups (about 10 ounces) fresh young spinach, washed, drained, and trimmed

1 small red onion, finely chopped

1½ cups halved cherry tomatoes

⅓ pound ricotta salata or Greek manouri cheese, cut into ½-inch cubes

½ cup pitted wrinkled black olives, such as Greek Thassos or Moroccan olives

The dressing

⅓ cup extra virgin olive oil

2 teaspoons sherry vinegar

2 teaspoons balsamic vinegar

2 teaspoons grainy Dijon mustard

1 teaspoon honey

½ teaspoon grated orange zest

Toast the pine nuts in a dry nonstick skillet over low heat for 4 to 5 minutes, stirring constantly, until lightly browned. Remove and set aside to cool.

Place the spinach in a serving bowl. Top with the onion, tomatoes, ricotta salata, olives, and pine nuts.

Whisk together all the dressing ingredients. Pour over the salad and serve.

PER SERVING: Calories 214; Fat 19g (Saturated 6g); Cholesterol 2mg; Sodium 460mg; Carbohydrates 10g; Fiber 3g (Digestible Carbohydrates 7g); Protein 5g.

Greek-Style Warm Broccoli Salad

Broccoli, like cauliflower, is usually blanched, boiled, or steamed and served as a warm salad in Greece. Embellishments are minimal—a little olive oil, freshly squeezed lemon juice, and herbs. I have added some nuts and feta to the dish, too.

8 servings

2 tablespoons pine nuts

2 pounds broccoli, trimmed and cut into florets

⅓ cup extra virgin olive oil

3 tablespoons fresh lemon juice

I garlic clove, finely chopped

I teaspoon chopped fresh basil

I teaspoon chopped flat-leaf parsley

I teaspoon chopped fresh mint

Salt and freshly ground black pepper

4 tablespoons crumbled Greek feta

Lightly toast the pine nuts in a dry nonstick skillet over low heat until pale golden, about 4 to 5 minutes. Remove from the skillet and set aside to cool.

Steam the broccoli for about 8 minutes and remove from the steamer.

In a medium bowl, whisk together the olive oil, lemon juice, garlic, basil, parsley, mint, and salt and pepper to taste. Place the broccoli in a serving bowl, toss with the dressing, and sprinkle with the pine nuts and feta. Serve immediately.

PER SERVING: Calories 137; Fat 11g (Saturated 2g); Cholesterol 4mg; Sodium 228mg; Carbohydrates 7g; Fiber 4g (Digestible Carbohydrates 3g); Protein 5g.

Spanish Mushroom Salad with Ham and Garlicky Dressing

Mushrooms are a low-carber's dream food: versatile, easy to pair with all sorts of other ingredients, filling, and carbless. In this salad the relatively neutral taste of the mushrooms is countered by the strong flavor of Spanish ham and by the robust flavors in the dressing, making it a lovely accompaniment to all kinds of grilled meats and omelets.

6 servings

---

8 ounces white button mushrooms, thinly sliced

2 teaspoons fresh lemon juice

2 slices Spanish ham, diced

The dressing

¼ cup extra virgin olive oil

1 teaspoon sherry vinegar

1 teaspoon Dijon mustard

1 small garlic clove, minced

½ teaspoon dried basil

½ teaspoon dried marjoram

½ teaspoon dried thyme

Salt and freshly ground black pepper

2 tablespoons grated aged Manchego or other hard sharp sheep's milk cheese

2 tablespoons flat-leaf parsley

Put the mushrooms in a salad bowl and toss with the lemon juice. Add the diced ham.

To make the dressing, in a medium bowl, whisk together the olive oil, vinegar, mustard, garlic, basil, marjoram, thyme, and salt and pepper to taste. Pour the dressing over the mushrooms. Add the cheese and 1 tablespoon parsley and toss gently. Garnish with remaining tablespoon parsley and serve.

PER SERVING: Calories 110; Fat 10g (Saturated 2g); Cholesterol 6mg; Sodium 339mg; Carbohydrates 2g; Fiber 1g (Digestible Carbohydrates 1g); Protein 3g.

Springtime Salads

Raw Artichoke Salad with Mint and Feta Vinaigrette

Artichokes are one of my all-time favorite vegetables. In the Mediterranean they come into season in the early spring, between mid- to late March and the end of April. In North America the season is a little later, but there is also a second harvest in the fall.

6 servings

I large lemon
12 young artichokes (see Note)
⅓ cup extra virgin olive oil
Strained juice of I large lemon
I garlic clove, minced
½ cup chopped fresh mint
Freshly ground black pepper
3 tablespoons crumbled Greek feta

Cut the lemon in half and squeeze it into a bowl filled with 3 to 4 cups water. Using a sharp paring knife, cut off the tough outer leaves and thorny top leaves from each artichoke. Cut the artichokes in half lengthwise and with a teaspoon scrape out any and all of the pinkish fuzz. Cut each half again in half lengthwise and drop immediately into the lemon water.

Place the olive oil, lemon juice, garlic, mint, pepper to taste, and feta in a blender and pulse together. Drain the artichokes from the lemon water, place in a bowl, add the feta vinaigrette, and toss. Serve immediately.

Note: You can also use frozen artichoke hearts for this dish, although the taste is nothing like that of fresh, in-season artichokes. If using frozen artichoke hearts, defrost them slowly from the freezer to the refrigerator and then add them to the marinade in step 2.

PER SERVING: Calories 156; Fat 13g (Saturated 2g); Cholesterol 4mg; Sodium 119mg; Carbohydrates 9g; Fiber 4g (Digestible Carbohydrates 5g); Protein 3g.

Fennel-Carrot Slaw with Capers and Cilantro

Although slaws are not part of the roster of Mediterranean salads, shredded raw vegetables, such as carrots and cabbage, appear in salads all over that part of the world. This salad is chock-full of Mediterranean ingredients and bespeaks one of the region's unifying characteristics: fresh, seasonal ingredients prepared simply but robustly.

6 servings

2 large fennel bulbs, trimmed

2 medium carrots

1 garlic clove, minced

2 tablespoons small capers in brine, drained

3 tablespoons chopped fresh cilantro

3 tablespoons extra virgin olive oil

Strained juice of 1 lemon

½ teaspoon ground ginger

Salt

Using a mandolin or knife, cut the fennel into thin ribbons, like matchsticks. Using a mandolin or grater, shred the carrots to the same thickness.

Toss the fennel, carrots, garlic, and capers together in a large bowl. Sprinkle with the cilantro.

Whisk together the olive oil, lemon juice, ginger, and salt. Pour over the salad, toss, and serve.

PER SERVING: Calories 97; Fat 7g (Saturated 1g); Cholesterol 0mg; Sodium 327mg; Carbohydrate 9g; Fiber 3g (Digestible Carbohydrates 6g); Protein 1g.

Romaine, Fennel, and Orange Salad

This salad takes its cue from a combination of flavors most common on the tables of Mediterranean Africa.

6 servings

1 small head romaine lettuce, cut into ½-inch strips

1 fennel bulb, stalks removed, quartered and thinly sliced

6 large radishes, halved and sliced

1 navel orange, skin and pith removed, flesh cut into 1-inch dice

½ cup snipped fresh dill

12 Moroccan olives, pitted

⅓ cup extra virgin olive oil

3 tablespoons sherry vinegar

½ teaspoon crushed fennel seeds

½ teaspoon rose peppercorns

Salt and freshly ground black pepper

Combine the lettuce, fennel, radishes, orange pieces, dill, and olives in a serving bowl.

In a medium bowl, whisk together the olive oil, vinegar, fennel seeds, peppercorns, and salt and pepper to taste. Pour over the salad, toss, and serve.

PER SERVING: Calories 162; Fat 14g (Saturated 2g); Cholesterol 0mg; Sodium 344mg; Carbohydrates 9g; Fiber 3g (Digestible Carbohydrates 6g); Protein 2g.

Salads Embellished with Seafood and Fish

Shrimp and Marinated Zucchini Salad

In the spring of 2004 in Greece, chefs all over Athens were making dishes with spaghetti-like strands of raw zucchini, like this one. The flavors are bright and refreshing, and the salad colorful and lovely to look at.

6 servings

2 medium zucchini

1 pound peeled and deveined cooked shrimp

⅓ cup extra virgin olive oil

4 tablespoons fresh strained lemon juice

1 garlic clove, pressed

1 tablespoon chopped fresh oregano

1 tablespoon chopped fresh mint

Salt and freshly ground black pepper

Trim the ends off the zucchini. Using a mandolin or a very sharp knife, cut the zucchini into paper-thin rounds.

Combine the zucchini with the shrimp in a large bowl.

In a medium bowl, whisk together the olive oil, lemon juice, garlic, oregano, mint, and salt and pepper to taste and pour the dressing over the zucchini and shrimp. Cover and marinate in the refrigerator for at least one hour and up to three. Serve chilled.

PER SERVING: Calories 194; Fat 13g (Saturated 2g); Cholesterol 147mg; Sodium 366mg; Carbohydrates 3g; Fiber 1g (Digestible Carbohydrates 2g); Protein 17g.

Tuna Salad with Arugula, Celery, and Roasted Peppers

This salad can easily be served as a main course, it's that filling.

8 salad servings

2 bunches arugula, trimmed and torn

2 celery ribs, finely chopped

1 small red onion, finely chopped

1 unpeeled hothouse cucumber, chopped

2 roasted red peppers, cored, seeded, and chopped

2 tablespoons chopped cilantro

2 tablespoons chopped fresh basil

2 tablespoons chopped flat-leaf parsley

4 tablespoons extra virgin olive oil

2 tablespoons balsamic vinegar

Salt and freshly ground black pepper

Two 6½-ounce cans good-quality white or albacore tuna in olive oil, drained very well
   and broken up with a fork

½ teaspoon ground dried thyme

1 teaspoon capers in brine, drained

Combine the arugula, celery, onion, cucumber, red peppers, cilantro, basil, and parsley in a large bowl. Drizzle with 3 tablespoons olive oil and the vinegar, season with salt and pepper to taste, and toss lightly.

Place the tuna over the salad, sprinkle with the thyme, and dot with the capers. Drizzle the remaining tablespoon olive oil over the tuna, toss again, and serve.

PER SERVING: Calories 120; Fat 8g (Saturated 1g); Cholesterol 15mg; Sodium 168mg; Carbohydrates 3g; Fiber 1g (Digestible Carbohydrates 2g); Protein 9g.

Marinated Octopus, Roasted Red Pepper, and Caper Salad

This recipe came about as collaboration between a friend and colleague, Christos Valtsoglou, owner of New York's Pylos restaurant, and me. Octopus is the quintessential Greek seafood, although it is popular all over the Mediterranean, especially in Spain and parts of southern Italy. I call for frozen octopus mainly because it is difficult to find fresh octopus in North America. I do not recommend what is commonly sold as sushi-quality octopus, which comes poached and skinned. Best to cook it from scratch.

6 servings

1 medium frozen octopus (about 3 pounds), defrosted

⅔ cup red wine vinegar

⅔ cup olive oil

1 garlic clove, slivered

1 teaspoon dried oregano

1 bay leaf

½ teaspoon whole black peppercorns

4 large roasted red peppers, seeded and coarsely chopped

4 scallions, white part only, thinly sliced

1 tablespoon minced fresh oregano

1 tablespoon minced flat-leaf parsley

3 tablespoons extra virgin olive oil, more if desired

3 small bunches frisée, trimmed

2 tablespoons small capers, rinsed and drained

Clean the octopus: Cut the octopus just below its eyes and remove the hood completely. Discard. Remove and discard the mouth and beak. Place the octopus in a large, heavy pot over high heat, cover, bring to a boil, reduce the heat to low, and cook for about 50 minutes, until it turns bright pink and is tender. Remove and cool. Peel off the purple membrane, if desired.

Cut the octopus into 8 tentacles and cut each tentacle at a slant into ½-inch oval slices.

In a medium bowl, whisk together the vinegar, ⅔ cup olive oil, garlic, dried oregano, bay leaf, and peppercorns. Place the octopus slices in a clean jar large enough to hold them and the marinade. Pour the marinade over the octopus. Cover and marinate for at least 24 hours or up to 1 week in the refrigerator.

To prepare the salad, combine the roasted red peppers and scallions in a large bowl. Remove the octopus from the marinade with a slotted spoon and add to the bowl. Add the fresh oregano, parsley, and 3 tablespoons extra virgin olive oil and stir to combine. Place the frisee on a large platter or divided among 6 individual plates. Spoon the salad on top, sprinkle with capers, and drizzle with additional extra virgin olive oil, if desired.

PER SERVING: Calories 296; Fat 7g (Saturated 1g); Cholesterol 145mg; Sodium 817mg; Carbohydrates 11g; Fiber 2g (Digestible Carbohydrates 9g); Protein 46g.

Cauliflower Salad with Shrimp, Cucumber, and Eggs

Cauliflower is the carte blanche vegetable for low-carb eaters, something to be used in pureed form as an imitator of buttery mashed spuds, something to be nibbled steamed or raw or stewed, mainly because it is virtually free of carbs, full of fiber, and filling to boot. A trick I learned from the late Bert Greene's Greene on Greens *is to steam or boil the cauliflower whole and then to cut it into florets. There is much less wasted that way; the florets stay whole and do not crumble into tiny specks, which so often happens when you cut them raw.*

8 servings

1 medium cauliflower (about 1½ pounds)

4 tablespoons extra virgin olive oil

2 tablespoons fresh lemon juice

Salt and freshly ground black pepper

2 teaspoons chopped fresh tarragon or 1 scant teaspoon dried

1 medium cucumber, peeled and cut into ⅛-inch rounds

16 Moroccan or Greek Thassos olives, pitted

2 hard-boiled eggs, quartered

16 medium shrimp peeled and deveined cooked shrimp

Remove the tough outer leaves of the cauliflower and as much of its hard, thick stem as possible without breaking the cauliflower into pieces. Place the cauliflower in a steaming basket inside a large pot filled with about 1½ to 2 inches of water, and steam it whole for 10 to 12 minutes, until tender but al dente. Drain when cool enough to handle and cut into florets. Place it in a large bowl.

Meanwhile, in a medium bowl, whisk together the olive oil, lemon juice, salt and pepper to taste, and tarragon. Pour two-thirds of the dressing over the warm cauliflower and toss to combine.

Add the cucumber and olives and toss gently. Place the quartered eggs and shrimp on top and drizzle with the remaining dressing. Serve immediately.

PER SERVING: Calories 124; Fat 10g (Saturated 2g); Cholesterol 75mg; Sodium 318mg; Carbohydrates 4g; Fiber 1g (Digestible Carbohydrates 3g); Protein 5g.

Spinach and Squid Salad

Here's a recipe that was inspired by a lovely salad created by a friend and chef, Yiannis Baxe-vannis, at his Athens restaurant, Hytra. It is slightly sweet thanks to the honey, the beets, and the carb-friendly raspberries, but still falls well within allowable carbohydrate rations. It's a delightful accompaniment to simple grilled meats and fish.

6 servings

1 large beet, scrubbed and trimmed

1 pound large squid, cleaned and cut into ½-inch rings

⅔ cup extra virgin olive oil

½ tablespoon Dijon mustard

1 teaspoon honey

3 tablespoons raspberry vinegar

1 tablespoon fresh orange juice

1 teaspoon grated orange zest

1 garlic clove, minced

Sea salt and freshly ground black pepper

1 pound baby spinach, stems trimmed

1 medium red onion, minced

½ pint raspberries, blueberries, or blackberries, chilled

Bring the beet to a boil in a small pot of salted water. Reduce heat and simmer for about 30 minutes, until tender but al dente. Drain and let cool. Using a vegetable peeler, pare the skin off the beet and cut off whatever remains of its root and stem ends. Using a mandolin or grater, grate the beets into matchstick-size pieces.

Bring a medium pot of salted water to a boil and blanch the squid for 3 minutes. Drain into a colander.

In a medium bowl, whisk together the olive oil, mustard, honey, vinegar, orange juice and zest, garlic, and salt and pepper to taste. Measure out half of the marinade and set aside.

Toss the squid with half the marinade. Cover and refrigerate for 1 to 3 hours. Place the beet in a small bowl and toss with a quarter of the marinade. Cover and refrigerate for 1 to 3 hours.

Assemble the salad on a large platter: Layer the spinach, followed by the beet and its marinade. Spread the onions on top, followed by the squid and its marinade. Drizzle with the remaining quarter of the marinade and toss in the berries. Serve immediately.

PER SERVING: Calories 274; Fat 18g (Saturated 3g); Cholesterol 176mg; Sodium 300mg; Carbohydrates 16g; Fiber 5g (Digestible Carbohydrates 11g); Protein 14g.

Salads with a Few Extra Carbs

Mediterranean Chicken and Wild Rice Salad

Wild rice, although not native to the Mediterranean, has found its way into the region's cupboards over the last decade or so. In Greece, where I live, it is—no pun intended—wildly popular, especially in restaurants. As I have opted to offer up slightly more than a handful of dishes with whole grains, I developed this salad. The earthiness of the wild rice counters the tart pungency of the marinated artichokes.

6 servings

½ cup wild rice, rinsed

3 tablespoons extra virgin olive oil

3 tablespoons tarragon vinegar

1 scant teaspoon dried tarragon

2 teaspoons Dijon mustard

Salt and freshly ground black pepper

3 cups cooked and shredded chicken

1 celery rib, finely chopped

½ cup chopped red onion

6 marinated artichoke hearts, drained and quartered

½ pound cherry tomatoes, halved

2 tablespoons tiny capers in brine, drained

Place the wild rice in a medium pot of salted water over medium-high heat. Bring to a boil, then reduce the heat and simmer until the rice is tender but al dente, about 35 minutes. Remove, drain in a colander, and rinse with cold water.

While the wild rice is boiling, whisk together 2 tablespoons of olive oil, the vinegar, tarragon, and mustard in a small bowl. Season with salt and pepper to taste. Place the chicken in a medium bowl and toss with half the dressing. Cover and let stand at room temperature for 20 minutes.

Heat the remaining olive oil in a small skillet, add the celery and onion, and sauté just until softened, about 3 minutes. Add the celery-onion mixture to the chicken. Add the wild rice, artichoke hearts, cherry tomatoes, and capers. Pour in the remaining dressing, toss gently, and serve.

PER SERVING: Calories 260; Fat 13g (Saturated 2g); Cholesterol 53mg; Sodium 428mg; Carbohydrates 16g; Fiber 2g (Digestible Carbohydrates 14g); Protein 20g.

Low-Carb Tabbouleh

I've included a handful of whole grains in this book—I just couldn't keep them out in light of the fact that the food here is all culled from the Mediterranean, where grains are so much a part of the diet. What makes this a low-carb tabbouleh is the relatively small amount of bulgur wheat, divided among 6 servings.

6 servings

½ cup bulgur wheat

2 ripe tomatoes, seeded and cut into ¼-inch dice

1 hothouse cucumber, peeled, seeded, and cut into ¼-inch dice

4 scallions, white part only, thinly sliced

1½ cups chopped flat-leaf parsley

½ cup chopped fresh mint

Salt

3 tablespoons extra virgin olive oil

2 to 3 tablespoons fresh lemon juice

½ teaspoon ground cinnamon

Pinch of allspice

1. Place the bulgur in a bowl. Cover with the tomatoes, then with the cucumber, followed by the scallions. Cover and let stand for 1 to 1½ hours.

2. Add the parsley, mint, salt to taste, olive oil, lemon juice, cinnamon, and allspice to the bulgur. Toss well, let stand for another 10 minutes, and serve.

PER SERVING: Calories 128; Fat 7g (Saturated 1g); Cholesterol 0mg; Sodium 212mg; Carbohydrates 15g; Fiber 5g (Digestible Carbohydrates 10g); Protein 3g.

Side Dish and Main Course Vegetables

I COULD HAVE JUST AS EASILY PLACED THE LITANY OF SIDE-dish vegetables in the salad chapter, since so many Mediterranean salads are really nothing more than cooked greens or boiled vegetables seasoned with olive oil and lemon juice or vinegar. I opted to place them here, side-by-side with main course vegetables, because to most Americans a "cooked" salad just isn't a salad.

The quality of vegetables in the Mediterranean is stellar, and from the souks of Morocco to the market stalls of Istanbul, shopping for one's vegetables, touching, squeezing, patting the very tomatoes, eggplants, zucchini, onions, and more that one is aiming to buy and cook is a way of life.

The role of vegetables on the table differs from place to place around the Mediterranean. In the Middle East and in Greece, for example, vegetables don't play second fiddle at table. There are countless recipes for main course vegetables, from hearty stews to luscious baked vegetable dishes to myriad stuffed vegetables. Many baked vegetable dishes contain cheese. Many of the classic vegetable stews contain starch either in the form of potatoes, rice, pasta, couscous, or bread, the latter meant to accompany many of these stews. For our purposes, obviously, I have omitted such dishes, although there are a few stews that might beg for a wedge of whole grain bread. There are, though, countless vegetable dishes that are perfectly suited to anyone watching his or her carbs.

In this chapter I have culled dishes from all over the region. Knowing that broccoli is a favorite vegetable among carb counters, I have included several of my favorite recipes. I believe that Italian cooks have the best broccoli dishes in the Mediterranean. I have included a few dishes for braised or otherwise cooked greens, and a couple of classic and not-so-classic stuffed vegetables, from the imam bayaldi—stuffed eggplant—that graces the tables of Turkey, Greece, and the Middle East, to newer dishes that take into account the specific needs of people watching their carbs. The tomatoes stuffed with cauliflower cream is one such creation, a dish in the Mediterranean style but not culled from tradition. The cinnamon-tinged stewed cauliflower, however, is a traditional dish, and one of the most unusual and simple vegetable stews of Greece.

This entire book is rife with vegetable-rich dishes. Many appear in other chapters, included in omelets, for example, in the chapter on eggs; in soups and small plates, and, of course, salads.

Horta

Boiled greens, the mainstay of the Greek diet for eons, are a no-brainer for the low-carber. A huge variety of greens is available, both in ethnic markets (especially Chinese markets) and in supermarkets and greengrocers, and, for the obsessed, online. The Greeks cooked their greens by bringing a pot of salted water to a boil, and then adding the greens, leaving the cover slightly askew, and cooking to desired tenderness. Greeks like their greens very well cooked. I prefer the texture of blanched greens more than boiled greens. In many cases, the boiling liquid can be cooled down, poured into a glass, spiked with a little lemon, and sipped. Traditional cooks know the greens juices are a panacea for all sorts of ailments.

Deciding whether to use bitter or sweet greens is a matter of taste. The most popular sweet greens are chard, collards, kale, beet greens, and sweet dandelion greens. In the bitter category, look for mustard greens, bitter dandelion greens, sorrel, and certain chicories.

Once cooked and drained, the greens are dressed in generous amounts of olive oil and either fresh lemon juice or vinegar. As a general rule among Greeks, lemon tends to be the favorite on sweet greens and vinegar is usually drizzled over bitter greens. You can boil the greens, drain them, and keep them in the refrigerator, undressed, for a few days before using. A half-pound of fresh greens, trimmed and boiled, is a good size portion for one.

Beet Greens Sizzled with Olive Oil and Garlic

Fresh spinach or chard work just as well. You can also add a handful of chopped prosciutto.

4 servings

1½ pounds fresh beet greens, trimmed

⅓ cup extra virgin olive oil

2 garlic cloves, slivered

Salt and freshly ground black pepper

2 to 3 tablespoons sherry or balsamic vinegar

4 tablespoons crumbled feta (optional)

Wash and dry the greens.

In a large, deep skillet or shallow, wide pot heat half of the olive oil over medium heat. Add the garlic and sauté until it softens, about 1 minute. Add the greens, and season with salt and pepper. Cover the skillet and let the greens steam in the oil for about 8 minutes until wilted. Remove the lid and continue cooking until most of the liquid has cooked off, another 6 to 7 minutes. Transfer the greens to a serving platter or individual plates. Add the remaining olive oil, the vinegar, and crumbled feta, and serve.

PER SERVING: Calories 196; Fat 18g (Saturated 2g); Cholesterol 0mg; Sodium 612mg; Carbohydrates 8g; Fiber 4g (Digestible Carbohydrates 4g); Protein 4g.

Sautéed Spinach with Bacon, Garlic, and White Wine

Sautéed spinach is an instant delicacy that matches well with almost all the main courses in this book.

4 servings

---

1 pound flat-leaf spinach
2 slices lean bacon, coarsely chopped
2 garlic cloves, thinly sliced
¼ cup dry white wine
Salt and freshly ground black pepper
2 tablespoons extra virgin olive oil

Trim the tough stems off the spinach but keep the leaves whole.

Heat the bacon in a large pot over medium heat. Add the garlic and cook, stirring, until softened, about 2 minutes. Add the spinach. Cover and cook for about 2 minutes, until slightly wilted. Remove the cover, stir, and raise the heat so that the juices from the spinach cook off. As soon as the spinach wilts to about half its volume, add the wine. Season with salt and pepper to taste. Continue cooking for about 10 minutes, or until tender. Remove from the heat, transfer to a serving platter, drizzle with the olive oil, and serve.

PER SERVING: Calories 110; Fat 8g (Saturated 1g); Cholesterol 7mg; Sodium 560mg; Carbohydrates 5g; Fiber 3g (Digestible Carbohydrates 2g); Protein 6g.

Braised Broccoli with Anchovies, Garlic, and Olive Oil

This dish, a southern Italian Christmas classic, can be made with either broccoli or broccoli rabe. It is traditionally sprinkled with toasted breadcrumbs, but I use toasted blanched almond slivers.

8 servings

3 salt-packed anchovies
⅓ cup skim milk or water
¼ cup blanched almond slivers
2 pounds broccoli, trimmed and cut into florets
Salt
¼ cup extra virgin olive oil
6 garlic cloves, halved
Freshly ground black pepper

Soak the anchovies in a small bowl with the milk for 1 hour. Drain and rinse very well, then chop them. Toast the almonds in a small, heavy skillet over low heat until lightly golden. Set aside to cool.

Bring a medium pot of salted water to a rolling boil and blanch the broccoli florets for about 4 minutes, until al dente. Drain.

Heat the olive oil in a large, heavy skillet over low heat, add the garlic, and sauté until it just begins to color, about 2 to 3 minutes. Add the anchovies to the skillet and mash together with the garlic. Cook for about 3 minutes, until the anchovies and garlic are one soft mass. Add the broccoli, cover the skillet, and cook for 5 to 6 minutes, until the broccoli is tender but not limp. Season with salt and generous pepper to taste. Remove from the heat, sprinkle with the toasted almonds, and serve.

Note: If using broccoli rabe, cut it into long stalks and trim them. Blanch it as you would the broccoli.

PER SERVING: Calories 160; Fat 11g (Saturated 2g); Cholesterol 15mg; Sodium 801mg; Carbohydrates 8g; Fiber 4g (Digestible Carbohydrates 4g); Protein 10g.

Sicilian "Drowned" Broccoli with Red Wine, Olives, Anchovies, and Provolone

This is one of the most unusual recipes for broccoli in all the Mediterranean, and admittedly one of the most visually unappealing! What it lacks in appearance it more than makes up for in complex, earthy flavors. Drowned broccoli is a traditional Christmas dish and it may be prepared with broccoli or broccoli rabe.

6 servings

8 anchovy fillets packed in salt

1½ cups skim milk or water

2 pounds broccoli

⅓ cup extra virgin olive oil

1 large onion, thinly sliced

⅓ cup finely chopped flat-leaf parsley

½ cup (about 3 ounces) sharp provolone, Greek Metsovone or Kasseri cheese,
    or Parmesan coarsely grated

½ cup finely chopped pitted Kalamata olives

½ cup dry red wine

Salt and freshly ground black pepper

Place the anchovy fillets in a small bowl with the milk to soak for about 30 minutes. Drain and rinse well.

Trim the toughest part of the stems off the broccoli and discard. Cut into florets and cut the remaining part of the stems into thin slices, about ¼-inch thick.

Heat the olive oil in a wide, shallow pot or large, deep skillet over medium heat, add the broccoli and onions and sauté for about 8 minutes. Add the parsley and cook for another 2 to 3 minutes.

Stir the cheese, olives, and wine into the broccoli. Cover, reduce the heat, and simmer for about 40 minutes, stirring occasionally, until there is no liquid left in the pot. If any liquid remains, remove the lid and continue simmering until the broccoli is very tender and the wine is completely cooked off. Season with salt and pepper to taste and serve.

PER SERVING: Calories 218; Fat 16g (Saturated 4g); Cholesterol 15mg; Sodium 469mg; Carbohydrates 13g; Fiber 5g (Digestible Carbohydrates 8g); Protein 10g.

Sautéed Broccoli with Garlic, Hot Pepper Flakes, and Pecorino

The first time I ever tasted this Italian classic was in the early 1980s, right about the time Italian cuisine began to shed its spaghetti-and-meatball aura in favor of higher things. I have been cooking it ever since.

6 servings

---

2 pounds broccoli or broccoli rabe
Salt
¼ cup extra virgin olive oil
6 garlic cloves, thinly sliced
½ teaspoon hot pepper flakes
⅓ cup freshly grated pecorino cheese
Salt and freshly ground black pepper

If using broccoli, trim the tough stem and cut into florets. If using broccoli rabe, peel off the tough bottom part of the stems. Bring a large pot of salted water to a rolling boil and blanch the broccoli for about 4 minutes until bright green or the broccoli rabe for about 2 minutes, until wilted. Remove and drain. Rinse immediately with very cold water. Drain again and pat dry. You can prepare the broccoli or broccoli rabe to this point up to a day ahead and store it in the refrigerator in a sealed plastic bag or container. Bring to room temperature before sautéing.

Heat the olive oil in a large, heavy skillet over medium heat, add the garlic and pepper flakes, and sauté for about 2 minutes, or until garlic is soft. Add the broccoli or broccoli rabe and continue sautéing for another 5 minutes, or until tender but al dente. Remove, toss with the cheese, sprinkle with salt and pepper to taste, and serve.

PER SERVING: Calories 136; Fat 10g (Saturated 2g); Cholesterol 2mg; Sodium 272mg; Carbohydrates 9g; Fiber 4g (Digestible Carbohydrates 5g); Protein 5g.

Braised Celery with Sharp Cheeses and Peppercorns

Celery and blue cheese or Roquefort are often served as an hors d'oeuvre, but the celery is braised, changing its character from clean and crisp to earthy and complex. This makes a lovely side dish to simple grilled meat preparations. I relish it on cold days.

4 side-dish servings

10 large celery stalks, bottoms and leaves trimmed
1 tablespoon extra virgin olive oil
1 tablespoon unsalted butter
1 small garlic clove, minced
¾ cup vegetable broth
2 tablespoons heavy cream
½ cup crumbled Roquefort or other blue cheese
¼ cup crumbled Greek feta
Freshly ground black pepper

Trim the celery and shave off any tough fibers with a vegetable peeler. Cut the celery into 2-inch pieces.

Heat the oil and butter in a medium skillet over medium heat. Raise the heat, add the celery, and cook until it begins to lightly caramelize, about 7 minutes. Add the garlic and stir. Pour in the vegetable broth, cover, reduce the heat to low, and cook for about 10 to 12 minutes, until tender.

Add the cream and crumbled cheeses. Season with pepper to taste. Raise the heat to medium and continue cooking, uncovered, until the cheese is melted and the sauce is thick, another 5 to 6 minutes. Serve hot.

PER SERVING: Calories 195; Fat 16g (Saturated 9g); Cholesterol 39mg; Sodium 582mg; Carbohydrates 8g; Fiber 3g (Digestible Carbohydrates 5g); Protein 6g.

My Greek Island
Summer Vegetable Medley

Yioula, the woman with whom I manned the stove for two grueling summers as an inexperienced restaurateur, showed me how to prepare this simple island dish. On our island of Ikaria, it is called soufico. *It is not unlike the Briam on page 38, but there is one main difference: In this dish all the vegetables are individually sautéed before being combined in one pot. Although this dish is very easy to make, it requires that you follow two golden rules: First, look for the absolute freshest ingredients and prepare the dish in summer when all that it calls for is in season; and second, have patience and go about preparing it slowly.*

6 main course servings

1 large eggplant, cut into $\frac{1}{4}$-inch rounds

2 large green peppers, cored, seeded, and cut into 1-inch strips

4 medium zucchini, cut into $\frac{1}{4}$-inch rounds

Salt

Extra virgin olive oil, as needed

1 large onion, finely chopped

3 garlic cloves, minced

1 medium potato, peeled and sliced into $\frac{1}{4}$-inch rounds

Freshly ground black pepper to taste

2 large, ripe tomatoes, grated

In 3 separate colanders, lightly salt the eggplant, peppers, and zucchini. Let drain for 1 hour. Wipe dry without washing.

Pour enough olive oil into a large skillet to come up the side $\frac{1}{4}$ inch. Place over medium heat, add the onion and garlic, and sauté until wilted, 6 to 7 minutes. Remove with a slotted spoon and set aside. Replenish the oil in the skillet if necessary. Add the potato slices and sauté lightly until their edges begin to color lightly.

Meanwhile, pour about ½ cup olive oil into a large, wide pot or rondeau. Remove the potatoes from the skillet with a slotted spoon and place in the pot, in 1, or at most, 2, layers. Season with a little salt and pepper and strew some of the onion-garlic mixture over the potatoes.

Next, lightly fry the zucchini in the same skillet, adding more olive oil if necessary. When lightly colored, remove with a slotted spoon and place over the potatoes, again in 1, or at most, 2, layers. Strew with some of the onion-garlic mixture. Do the same with the eggplant, replenishing the oil in the skillet if necessary. Again, sprinkle with some of the onion-garlic mixture. Next, fry the peppers, ever so lightly, just to soften. Place over the eggplant slices. Season with a little pepper. Add the grated tomato. Cover and simmer for 20 to 30 minutes, until the vegetables are very tender and almost melded together in a kind of one-pot napoleon.

PER SERVING: Calories 216; Fat 12g (Saturated 2g); Cholesterol 0mg; Sodium 210mg; Carbohydrates 26g; Fiber 8g (Digestible Carbohydrates 18g); Protein 5g.

Summer Greens and Purslane Stewed with Zucchini and Garlic

Here's a simple recipe that speaks of the innate healthfulness of the Mediterranean and of the importance of seasonality. Purslane, a summer green that runs rampant in backyards and gardens all over the Mediterranean as well as all over North America, is one of the world's most healthful weeds! Its succulent leaves have an almost imperceptible, lovely sour taste a little reminiscent of lime. Purslane is filled with nutrients and is especially rich in antioxidants. It is eaten raw in salads and also cooked, as in this typical Greek island recipe.

6 side-dish servings

⅓ cup extra virgin olive oil

1 large red onion, chopped

3 garlic cloves, minced

2 pounds amaranth greens or Swiss chard, tough stems trimmed

1½ pounds purslane, trimmed

2 large ripe tomatoes, grated or peeled and chopped (you don't have to seed them—
   Greeks never do)

6 small zucchini, trimmed

Juice of 2 lemons

Salt and freshly ground black pepper

Heat the olive oil in a large pot over medium heat. Add the onion and garlic and cook until wilted. Add the amaranth and purslane, cover, and wilt. Add the tomatoes and 1 cup water. With the lid ajar, simmer until most of the liquid has evaporated, about 12 minutes.

Add the whole zucchini and lemon juice. Season with salt and pepper to taste. Simmer for another 6 to 8 minutes, until the zucchini is tender. Serve warm or at room temperature.

PER SERVING: Calories 206; Fat 13g (Saturated 2g); Cholesterol 0mg; Sodium 280mg; Carbohydrates 22g; Fiber 7g (Digestible Carbohydrates 15g); Protein 7g.

Braised Green Beans with Garlic and Herbs

Green beans are mainstay of the summer diet in most of the countries around the Mediterranean Basin. The Greeks and Turks love their green bean stews; the Italians prefer bean dishes that are more al dente. Here's a recipe that borrows from both traditions.

8 side-dish servings

Salt

2 pounds fresh string beans, trimmed

1 tablespoon unsalted butter

1 tablespoon extra virgin olive oil

6 large garlic cloves, smashed

2 medium ripe tomatoes, peeled and diced, with their juices reserved

Freshly ground black pepper

½ cup chopped fresh basil

2 tablespoons chopped fresh thyme

Bring a large pot of salted water to a rolling boil and blanch the beans for 3 minutes. Drain the beans in a colander and rinse them under cold running water.

In a large, wide pot or deep skillet heat the butter and olive oil together. Add the garlic. Cover and cook over very low heat for about 15 minutes, stirring occasionally, until the garlic becomes golden. Do not let it burn. Add the tomatoes. Uncover, raise the heat to medium, and let some of the tomato juices boil off.

Add the green beans and toss to coat. Season with salt and pepper to taste. Reduce the heat to low, cover, and cook for about 10 more minutes, or until the beans are tender. Add the basil and thyme, toss, and cook, covered, for another 2 to 3 minutes, or until the herbs have wilted. Remove from the heat and serve.

PER SERVING: Calories 79; Fat 4g (Saturated 1g); Cholesterol 4mg; Sodium 415mg; Carbohydrates 12g; Fiber 4g (Digestible Carbohydrates 8g); Protein 3g.

Cinnamon-Scented Cauliflower Stew

Cauliflower is one of those vegetables that incite either ire or awe. Ire because of its malodorous steam as it cooks; awe because of its healthfulness and versatility. Cauliflower contains all sorts of good nutrients, from a hefty dose of vitamins A and C to potassium and folic acid.

6 servings

6 sun-dried tomatoes, drained if packed in oil

2 tablespoons extra virgin olive oil

1 cup finely chopped red onion

2 garlic cloves, finely chopped

1 medium cauliflower (2 pounds), trimmed and cut into florets

1 cup chopped plum tomatoes, with their juices

2 bay leaves

1 cinnamon stick

One 1-inch piece orange zest

Salt and freshly ground black pepper

12 cracked green olives, pitted, rinsed, and drained

2 tablespoons chopped flat-leaf parsley

Place the sun-dried tomatoes in a bowl with 1 cup of warm water to soak for 1 hour. Remove, drain, coarsely chop, reserve the water, and set aside.

Heat 3 tablespoons olive oil in a large, wide pot over medium heat, add the onion and garlic and cook, stirring, until wilted, about 8 minutes.

Add the cauliflower florets, toss to coat in the oil, then add the tomatoes. Stir gently. Add enough water to come about three-quarters of the way up the cauliflower. Add the bay leaves, cinnamon, and orange zest. Season lightly with salt and pepper. Reduce the heat to low, cover, and simmer for 20 minutes.

Add the sun-dried tomatoes. Cook another 5 minutes, then add the olives. Stir gently. Cook another 5 minutes for the olives to warm through and the flavors to meld. Taste for seasoning, add salt and pepper accordingly, and stir in the parsley. Remove the bay leaves, cinnamon, and orange zest and serve, either hot or at room temperature.

PER SERVING: Calories 115; Fat 7g (Saturated 1g); Cholesterol 0mg; Sodium 481mg; Carbohydrates 12g; Fiber 5g (Digestible Carbohydrates 7g); Protein 4g.

Tomatoes Stuffed with Pureed Cauliflower and Feta

It took me a while to get used to the idea of making a stuffed tomato dish that did not include rice, since in Greece, stuffed tomatoes tend to mean but one specific rice-filled aromatic dish. I forfeited all my own preconceptions and went ahead with something at once unusual but also elusively Mediterranean.

8 servings

8 medium ripe tomatoes

1 small cauliflower (about ½ pound), trimmed and cut into florets

Salt

2 tablespoons extra virgin olive oil

4 tablespoons creamy Greek feta, crumbled

⅓ pound skim-milk ricotta

2 teaspoons dried mint

3 tablespoons light cream

2 tablespoons fresh lemon juice

1 large egg

Freshly ground black pepper

Preheat the oven to 350°F. Lightly oil an ovenproof glass baking dish large enough to hold the tomatoes snugly in 1 layer.

Cut the crowns off the tomatoes and set aside. Carefully scoop out the pulp without puncturing the tomato skins. Place the pulp in a food processor. Salt the tomatoes lightly on the inside and set aside upside down on a tray lined with paper towels to drain.

Bring a medium pot of salted water to a rolling boil and blanch the cauliflower until soft, about 8 minutes. Remove and drain in a colander.

Add the cooked cauliflower to the tomato pulp and olive oil in the food processor. Process until just pureed. Add the feta, ricotta, and mint and pulse to combine. Add the cream in tablespoon increments, pulsing on and off until the mixture is smooth and creamy. Add the lemon juice and then the egg, pulsing after each addition. Add pepper to taste.

Fill each tomato with the cauliflower mixture. Place the caps gently back on the tomatoes without pressing down. Place in the baking pan, cover with aluminum foil, and bake for about 40 minutes, until the tomatoes are tender and the filling is set. Remove from the oven, cool slightly, and serve. This goes great with any of the greens dishes and with most of the broccoli dishes. For a slightly more decorative touch, try serving the tomatoes on small beds of boiled greens.

PER SERVING: Calories 103; Fat 7g (Saturated 2g); Cholesterol 38mg; Sodium 302mg; Carbohydrates 7g; Fiber 2g (Digestible Carbohydrates 5g); Protein 4g.

Imam Bayaldi

The name of this dish means "the imam (priest) fainted." It's both a Turkish and Greek favorite, and its name is meant to show just how good it is.

8 main course servings

3 tablespoons olive oil

4 medium red onions, coarsely chopped

2 garlic cloves, minced

1½ cups coarsely chopped plum tomatoes, with their juices

¼ cup red wine

16 Kalamata olives, pitted, rinsed, and coarsely chopped

Salt and freshly ground black pepper

⅔ cup finely chopped flat-leaf parsley

⅔ cup finely chopped fresh mint

½ cup finely chopped fresh oregano

4 medium eggplants, halved

Salt

Olive oil for brushing the eggplants

Preheat the broiler. Prepare the filling: In a large heavy skillet heat the olive oil over medium heat. Add the onions and garlic. Cover, reduce the heat to low, and let the mixture steam in the oil until soft and lightly colored, 12 to 15 minutes, stirring occasionally. Add the tomatoes, raise the heat, and bring to a simmer. Pour in the wine. As soon as the wine steams off, reduce the heat and simmer with the cover slightly ajar, until there is no longer any liquid in the pan from the tomatoes. Five minutes before removing, add the olives and season with salt and pepper to taste. Remove from the heat and cool slightly. Toss in the parsley, mint, and oregano.

Meanwhile, prepare the eggplants: Brush generously on both sides with olive oil and place cut side up on a lightly oiled shallow baking pan. The eggplants should glisten from the oil. Place the pan on a rack 8 inches from the heat source and bake until the flesh is softened, 10 to 12 minutes. Turn and repeat on the other side for about 5 minutes, until softened. The eggplant should not be fully cooked. Take care, too, not to char the eggplants; that's why it's important for them to cook at a distance from the broiler. Remove and cool slightly. Turn the oven to 350° F.

Scrape out as much of the pulp as possible without puncturing the eggplant. Chop the pulp and mix it in with the onion mixture. Taste and season with additional salt and pepper as needed. Fill the eggplants with the onion mixture, forming a rounded mound in each half. Place on a lightly oiled baking sheet and bake for about 30 minutes, until the eggplant is completely soft and the flavors have melded together.

PER SERVING: Calories 142; Fat 8g (Saturated 1g); Cholesterol 0mg; Sodium 426mg; Carbohydrates 17g; Fiber 6g (Digestible Carbohydrates 11g); Protein 3g.

Portobello "Pizza" Margherita

Portobellos are a fairly recent addition to the gamut of commercially available mushrooms throughout the Mediterranean. This dish came about as a lark, one night at home, with two kids clamoring for pizza, and Mom not in the mood or mode to deal with dough.

6 servings

6 large portobello mushrooms, 4 to 5 inches in diameter

3 teaspoons extra virgin olive oil

6 teaspoons grated Parmesan

1 cup plus 2 tablespoons tomato sauce

18 fresh basil leaves

Salt and freshly ground black pepper

6 heaping tablespoons shredded mozzarella

Preheat the oven to 375°F. Lightly oil a shallow baking pan large enough to fit the portobellos in 1 layer.

Carefully remove the stems from the mushrooms and either discard or save for another use. Using a teaspoon, scrape the black fan-like ridges off the underside of the mushrooms, taking care not the break the caps.

Brush each mushroom with ½ teaspoon olive oil and place on the baking dish, cap side down. Sprinkle each with 1 teaspoon Parmesan and spread 3 tablespoons tomato sauce over each mushroom. Place 3 basil leaves on each mushroom and season with salt and pepper to taste. Sprinkle 3 tablespoons mozzarella over each mushroom. Bake until the cheese melts and the mushrooms are firm but tender, about 15 minutes. Remove from the oven and serve immediately.

PER SERVING: Calories 121; Fat 6g (Saturated 2g); Cholesterol 10mg; Sodium 603mg; Carbohydrates 8g; Fiber 2g (Digestible Carbohydrates 6g); Protein 6g.

The Mediterranean Soup Kitchen

W HILE ALMOST EVERY COUNTRY IN THE MEDITER-
ranean can count a number of similar lamb or vegetable dishes, for example, soups all have their own
highly nationalistic character. Chicken soup with egg-lemon sauce
is associated with Greece and nowhere else; Harira is Moroccan,
period. Ditto for almost all the soups simmering on stovetops from
Istanbul to Tangiers. The one thing all Mediterranean soup cookery has in common, though, is its adherence to seasonality. Vegetable soups are made when specific vegetables are in season; meat
soups generally belong to the domain of winter; fish soups have
their season, too, depending on the catch.

As a Greek, inured to a cuisine that shares more with its eastern
neighbors than with Mediterranean countries further west, soup,
although not a mainstay of the table, is almost always served as a
main course. Greek soups, like those of the Middle East, are meals

in themselves. Sometimes there is little to distinguish a soup from a stew beyond the amount of liquid in the pot. Greece also shares a certain snobbery with some Middle Eastern countries toward soups. I have many friends who consider soup, regardless how filling it may be, not quite sating since you can't cut it with a knife. There is also a certain connotation that soup is poor man's food.

The one exception is fish soup. Certainly in Greece, but also in other places along the Mediterranean coast, fish soup is a delicacy and a much revered tradition. In Greece alone, there are dozens of different recipes for fish and seafood soups, some with vegetables and herbs, others enriched with dark barley rusks, others thickened with a little rice and an egg-lemon liaison. From the classic bouillabaisse (not included here because it is not something people make readily at home) to saffron-scented soups from other places, such as Spain, to simple Italian seafood soups, the sea and its treasures have always figured prominently in the Mediterranean soup pot.

Cream soups are, of course, the domaine of the French and seldom found in other parts of the Mediterranean. I have included two here: a French cream of mushroom soup and a delicious cream of cauliflower soup served with a dollop of roe, which is a Franco-Grecque recipe of mine.

In other recipes, it took some tinkering with a handful of the more traditional dishes to make them appropriate for those watching their carb intake, since so many Mediterranean soups contain ingredients meant to make them substantial, from legumes and potatoes, to pasta and rice. In some soups I have bowed to the Mediterranean's love affair with these ingredients and have used them in small quantities, thus limiting the total carbohydrate intake per serving.

Still, there are enough soups with few or no carbs throughout the Mediterranean to fill an entire book. For example, vegetable soups abound. One of my favorites is the Turkish roasted eggplant soup. It has everything: a rich, substantial texture, facility of preparation, and great flavor. Another favorite is a modern roasted red pepper soup that I often serve at dinner parties. It is not traditional but it looks and tastes great. Chicken and other meat soups abound, too, and I have included some of my own favorite chicken soups.

Most of the soups in this chapter may be eaten either as a first course or as a main course.

Vegetable Soups

Italian Spinach Soup with Brown Rice and Parmesan

Mediterranean comfort foods almost inevitably call for some type of grain, and in the less austere low-carb diets whole grains are permitted with measure. This is a homey Italian soup, perfect for cold winter nights and lazy weekends.

8 servings

1 tablespoon extra virgin olive oil, plus 4 teaspoons for drizzling

1 large onion, finely chopped

2 garlic cloves, minced

3 pounds fresh spinach, trimmed and finely chopped

8 cups chicken or beef broth

½ cup brown rice

Salt and freshly ground black pepper

8 teaspoons grated Parmesan

Heat the olive oil in a soup pot over medium heat and add the onion and garlic. Reduce the heat to low and cook, stirring, until soft about 5 minutes. Add the spinach and stir to coat in the oil. Cover the pot and cook the spinach until reduced to about one third of its volume.

Using a slotted spoon, remove the spinach and onions from the pot, leaving the liquid. Place the spinach mixture in a food processor and puree until smooth, then return it to the pot. Pour in the broth and stir. Raise the heat and bring to a boil. Add the rice. As soon as the soup comes to a boil, reduce the heat and simmer until the rice is cooked, about 40 minutes. Season with salt and pepper to taste. Serve in individual bowls drizzled with ½ teaspoon olive oil and sprinkled with 1 teaspoon Parmesan.

PER SERVING: Calories 164; Fat 9g (Saturated 2g); Cholesterol 6mg; Sodium 1,124mg; Carbohydrates 16g; Fiber 4g (Digestible Carbohydrates 12g); Protein 7g.

Leek, Fennel, and Celery Soup
with Sautéed Shrimp

This soup is both wintry and bright. The flavors are delicate and work well with any number of dishes in the book, from the cooked greens salads to various fish dishes—it's great as a starter with whole fish baked in salt, for example. It's also a light and subtle foil to heartier fare, such as any of the roasted chicken dishes.

6 servings

2 tablespoons extra virgin olive oil

1 leek, whites and tender greens, coarsely chopped (about 2 cups)

1 medium fennel bulb, trimmed and coarsely chopped (about 2 cups)

1 cup coarsely chopped celery

Salt and freshly ground black pepper

1 teaspoon finely ground fennel seeds

4 cups vegetable broth

½ pound medium shrimp, peeled and deveined

1 small garlic clove, crushed but kept whole

1 tablespoon ouzo

¼ cup heavy cream

1 teaspoon fresh lemon juice

Heat 1 tablespoon olive oil in a medium soup pot over medium heat. Add the chopped leek, fennel, and celery and cook, stirring occasionally until the vegetables begin to caramelize lightly, about 15 minutes. Season with salt and pepper to taste and the ground fennel, stir, and pour in the broth. Bring to a boil, reduce the heat, cover, and simmer for 20 to 25 minutes, until the vegetables are very soft.

Remove from heat. Using a slotted spoon, remove about three-quarters of the vegetables from the pot and place in a food processor. Puree, then place back in the pot.

Heat the remaining tablespoon of olive oil in a medium nonstick skillet, add the shrimp and garlic and season lightly with salt and pepper. Sauté until the shrimp turns bright pink and slightly browned around the edges. Pour in the ouzo and steam it off.

Remove the garlic clove from the skillet. Add the shrimp and their pan juices to the soup. Heat. Pour in the cream and continue cooking until warmed through. Stir in the lemon juice and serve.

PER SERVING: Calories 146; Fat 9g (Saturated 3g); Cholesterol 70mg; Sodium 654mg; Carbohydrates 10g; Fiber 2g (Digestible Carbohydrates 8g); Protein 7g.

Turkish Grilled Eggplant Soup

To my Greek friends, inured to savoring roasted eggplants in the form of a dip, this soup always comes as a surprise.

8 servings

3 large eggplants

2 large ripe tomatoes, halved

1 medium red onion, quartered

1 small head of garlic

Salt

1 teaspoon dried thyme

6 tablespoons extra virgin olive oil

5 cups chicken broth

Freshly ground black pepper

⅓ cup heavy cream

1 tablespoon fresh mint leaves, cut into thin strips, for garnish

Light the broiler or grill. Roast the eggplants about 6 inches from the heat source, turning, until charred and soft all over. This will take about 40 minutes. You can also grill the eggplants on top of the stove over a low flame or burner.

If you prepare the eggplants on top of the stove or grill them on a barbecue, you can roast the tomatoes, onion, and garlic simultaneously: Preheat the oven to 350°F and lightly oil a baking pan. Quarter the tomatoes and the onion. Wrap the garlic in aluminum foil. Place the tomatoes and onion in the baking pan and place the garlic on the bottom of the oven. Sprinkle the tomatoes with salt and thyme. Bake until the vegetables are lightly charred, about 30 minutes. Remove from the oven and set aside.

Remove the eggplants from the grill or stovetop and let stand until cool enough to handle. Cut lengthwise down the middle, scoop out the pulp, leaving behind the denser, most compact part of the seeds. Place the pulp in a food processor and add the tomatoes and onion. Unwrap the garlic and squeeze the pulp into the food processor. Process, adding enough of the olive oil in a slow, steady stream until the mixture becomes a very smooth puree.

Place the chicken broth in a medium soup pot over medium heat and bring to a simmer. Add the eggplant puree and cook, stirring, until smooth and evenly distributed and the flavors meld, about 10 minutes. Season with a little salt and pepper. Pour in the cream, lower the heat, and cook, stirring, until the soup is smooth and velvety, about 3 to 4 minutes. Serve in individual bowls and sprinkle each with a few strands of mint.

PER SERVING: Calories 217; Fat 16g (Saturated 0g); Cholesterol 13mg; Sodium 787mg; Carbohydrates 18g; Fiber 6g (Digestible Carbohydrates 12g); Protein 3g.

Cold Roasted Pepper Soup with Feta Cream

Roasted pepper soup is the invention of Mediterranean-minded American cooks who more than a decade ago fell in love with the sweet, unctuous roasted red pepper and have since adapted it to many dishes. Greeks often serve roasted red peppers garnished with a sprinkling of crumbled feta. The pleasantly sour taste of the cheese makes a bold contrast to the sweetness of the soup.

6 servings

10 red peppers, roasted, peeled, cored, and seeded

2 chiles, roasted, peeled, and seeded

2 tablespoons extra virgin olive oil

1 medium red onion, finely chopped

4 large garlic cloves, minced

2 teaspoons finely chopped fresh oregano

6 cups chicken or vegetable broth

Salt and freshly ground black pepper

2 tablespoons fresh strained lemon juice

⅓ cup light cream

The Feta Cream

3 tablespoons crumbled Greek feta

2 teaspoons extra virgin olive oil

1 teaspoon fresh strained lemon juice

1 tablespoons chopped fresh mint

Freshly ground black pepper

Place the peppers and chiles in a food processor and puree until smooth.

Heat the olive oil in a large, heavy soup pot over medium heat, add the onion and garlic and sauté, stirring, until soft and translucent, about 7 minutes. Add the pepper puree and oregano and stir. Pour in the broth and bring to a boil. Season with salt and pepper to taste. Reduce the heat and simmer for 15 minutes. Add the lemon juice and stir. Add the cream, stir to combine well, and simmer another 5 minutes, or until smooth. Remove from heat. You can serve the soup at this point or chill it and serve cold.

To make the Feta Cream, place the feta, olive oil, lemon juice, mint, and pepper to taste in a food processor and pulse until smooth. Serve the soup, either hot or cold, with a little of the Feta Cream spooned into each bowl. You can also put the Feta Cream in a pastry bag and decoratively pipe it into each bowl.

PER SERVING: Calories 221; Fat 16g (Saturated 6g); Cholesterol 27mg; Sodium 1,056mg; Carbohydrates 17g; Fiber 5g (Digestible Carbohydrates 12g); Protein 4g.

Fresh Tomato Soup with Moroccan Spices

With tomatoes as good as they are all over the Mediterranean, it stands to reason that myriad dishes have evolved from one end of the basin to the other. The French have their cream of tomato soups, the Spanish their gazpacho, the Greeks their tomato and bulgur wheat soups, and more. I especially like Moroccan tomato soups that couple the summer's quintessential vegetable with densely aromatic spices. The balance is lovely.

6 servings

---

8 large ripe tomatoes, seeded and coarsely chopped

2 tablespoons extra virgin olive oil

1 large yellow onion, coarsely chopped

1 teaspoon paprika

1 scant teaspoon finely chopped fresh ginger

1 scant teaspoon ground cumin

1 cinnamon stick

1 teaspoon honey

2 cups chicken broth

3 tablespoons chopped flat-leaf parsley

2 tablespoons chopped cilantro

1 tablespoon fresh lemon juice

Place the tomatoes in a food processor and puree. Set aside.

Heat the olive oil in a large soup pot over medium heat, add the onion, and cook until wilted, about 8 minutes. Add the paprika, ginger, cumin, and cinnamon and stir to coat. Pour in the tomatoes, honey, broth, and half the parsley and cilantro. Raise the heat and bring the soup to a boil, then reduce the heat and simmer, partially covered, for 20 minutes, or until slightly thickened. Remove from the heat, cool to room temperature, and chill for 2 to 3 hours before serving. Just before serving stir in the lemon juice and remaining parsley and cilantro.

PER SERVING: Calories 122; Fat 7g (Saturated 1g); Cholesterol 2mg; Sodium 358mg; Carbohydrates 15g; Fiber 3g (Digestible Carbohydrates 12g); Protein 3g.

Cream of Cauliflower Soup
with Salmon Roe or Caviar

A few years ago I dined on a velouté of cauliflower with caviar at the French Laundry in Napa. It's one of the dishes I have eaten in my twenty-odd years of professional restaurant-going that I will never forget. I borrowed the idea, originally serving my version of the soup with bottargo, the pressed roe of either tuna or mullet that is considered a delicacy in the Mediterranean. Feel free to use it here, too, although it is as pricey as the best caviar. This rendition calls for either salmon roe or one of the less expensive caviars.

8 servings

---

1 tablespoon unsalted butter

1 large red onion, minced

2 large garlic cloves, minced

1 large cauliflower, finely chopped

1 scant teaspoon curry powder

2 cups skim milk

6 cups chicken or vegetable broth

Salt and freshly ground black pepper

½ cup evaporated skim milk

2 tablespoons fresh lemon juice

8 scant teaspoons salmon roe or caviar

8 teaspoons extra virgin olive oil for drizzling

Heat the butter in a large soup pot over medium heat. Add the onion and garlic and cook until wilted and lightly golden. Add the cauliflower and toss to coat. Sprinkle in the curry and stir. Pour in the milk and broth, raise the heat, and bring to a boil. Reduce the heat, season with salt and pepper to taste, and simmer for 30 to 35 minutes, until the cauliflower is very tender. Skim off the top of the soup as it simmers.

Strain the soup into a large bowl, reserving the liquid. Place the vegetables in a food processor and process to a very smooth puree. Return the liquid and puree back to the pot. Bring back to a boil over medium heat. Add the evaporated milk and cook, stirring for 5 minutes to thicken. Stir in the lemon juice. Just before removing the soup from heat, stir in the remaining tablespoon butter.

Ladle the soup into individual bowls. Place 1 scant teaspoon salmon roe or caviar on each individual serving spoon and place the spoon in the bowl. Drizzle 1 teaspoon olive oil over the surface of each bowl and sprinkle with freshly ground pepper.

PER SERVING: Calories 164; Fat 10g (Saturated 3g); Cholesterol 28mg; Sodium 977mg; Carbohydrates 13g; Fiber 3g (Digestible Carbohydrates 10g); Protein 7g.

Velvety Mushroom Soup with Red Wine and Cream

This is a pretty classic cream of mushroom soup, easy to make, easy to serve, versatile, festive, but also simple enough to make frequently.

6 servings

2 ounces dried porcini
2 ounces dried morels
½ pound portobello mushrooms
½ pound cultivated button mushrooms
1 tablespoon extra virgin olive oil
1 teaspoon unsalted butter
3 shallots, finely chopped
2 garlic cloves, pressed
½ cup finely chopped flat-leaf parsley
1 teaspoon finely chopped fresh thyme
⅓ cup dry red wine
4 cups vegetable or chicken broth
Salt and freshly ground black pepper
⅓ cup heavy cream

Place the porcini and morels in 2 small separate bowls and pour in just enough warm water to cover. Set aside for 30 minutes to soften. Drain, reserve the water, and drain again through a fine-mesh sieve or cheesecloth to trap any dirt or sand. Set aside.

Rinse the portobellos and cultivated mushrooms quickly under cold water, pat dry, and chop them.

Heat the olive oil and butter in a large pot over high heat, add the shallots, garlic, parsley, and thyme and sauté for 2 minutes, stirring. Add the portobellos and cultivated mushrooms and stir to coat. Add the porcini and morels and stir. Pour in the wine, raise the heat, and as soon as the wine steams up, add the broth and mushroom water. Bring to a boil, season with salt and pepper to taste, reduce the heat to medium, and simmer for 7 to 8 minutes, until the mushrooms are tender.

Using a slotted spoon, remove about half of the solids, place in a food processor, and puree until smooth. Return to the pot and the heat. Add the cream and stir. Cook for another 5 minutes, until the soup thickens slightly. Remove from heat and serve.

PER SERVING: Calories 180; Fat 9g (Saturated 4g); Cholesterol 20mg; Sodium 881mg; Carbohydrates 16g; Fiber 4g (Digestible Carbohydrates 12g); Protein 9g.

Greek Salad Gazpacho
with Kalamata Olive Croutons

Greek salad gazpacho is my nod to the fusion fever that has taken over the Mediterranean during the last few years. The soup is a great starter with grilled meats and some of the heartier salads in this book, as well as with the robust shrimp recipes. You can use any black olive paste to make the croutons if you can't specifically find Kalamala olive paste.

8 servings

The Kalamata Olive Croutons

Two 1-inch slices day-old rye or whole-grain bread, cut into 1-inch cubes

2 tablespoons Kalamata olive paste

1 tablespoon extra virgin olive oil

The Soup

8 large ripe tomatoes, coarsely chopped

2 large green peppers, cored, seeded, and coarsely chopped

1 fresh green or red chile, seeded and coarsely chopped

1 large red onion, coarsely chopped

1 large unpeeled seedless cucumber, coarsely chopped

2 garlic cloves, minced

1 tablespoon chopped fresh oregano

1½ cups tomato juice

2 tablespoons extra virgin olive oil

2 tablespoons fresh strained lemon juice

Salt and freshly ground white pepper

Preheat the oven to 325°F. Lightly oil a small sheet pan. Toss the cubed bread, olive paste, and olive oil together in a medium bowl. Arrange on the sheet pan and bake for about 25 minutes, until crisp. Remove and set aside to cool.

To make the soup, place the tomatoes, pepper, chile, onion, cucumber, and garlic in a food processor and puree. Add the oregano and pulse to combine. Transfer to a bowl and stir in the tomato juice, olive oil, and lemon juice. Season with salt and pepper to taste and chill for at least 2 hours but not more than 4. Serve in individual bowls, dividing the croutons to evenly top each bowl.

PER SERVING: Calories 155; Fat 8g (Saturated 1g); Cholesterol 0mg; Sodium 489mg; Carbohydrates 21g; Fiber 5g (Digestible Carbohydrates 16g); Protein 4g.

Greens and Lentil Soup with Bacon and Olive Paste

I developed a similar soup for Pylos restaurant in New York City, omitting the bacon and using a whole head of roasted garlic. The bacon here gives this soup some added texture, and lentil soups are one of the classic soul-warmers of the Mediterranean.

8 servings

1 pound Swiss chard, tough stems removed and discarded

1 pound fresh spinach, trimmed

5 tablespoons extra virgin olive oil

1 slice lean bacon, coarsely chopped

1 medium red onion, minced

2 garlic cloves, minced

4 ounces small brown lentils, rinsed well

6 cups vegetable broth

1 bay leaf

3 sprigs fresh oregano

2 tablespoons tomato paste

3 tablespoons sherry vinegar

Salt and freshly ground black pepper

2 tablespoons Kalamata olive paste

Coarsely chop the chard and spinach and wash well. Set aside.

Heat 3 tablespoons olive oil in a large soup pot over medium heat and add the bacon. Cook, stirring until lightly browned. Add the onion and cook until soft, about 7 minutes. Add the garlic and cook for 1 minute. Add the lentils and stir to coat.

Empty the greens into the pot. Cover and allow them to wilt. Add the broth, raise the heat, and bring to a boil. Add the bay leaf and oregano, reduce the heat, and simmer until the lentils and greens are very tender, about 30 minutes. Add the tomato paste and stir to combine. Add the vinegar, season with salt and pepper to taste, and simmer another 5 minutes. Mix in the olive paste and remaining 2 tablespoons olive oil and serve.

PER SERVING: Calories 221; Fat 8g (Saturated 1g); Cholesterol 2mg; Sodium 1,127mg; Carbohydrates 28g; Fiber 10g (Digestible Carbohydrates 18g); Protein 13g.

Soups with Meat

Chicken and Vegetable Soup
with Brown Rice and Fennel

This soup, seasoned with Italian herbs, is filling thanks to the small amount of brown rice. It can easily be served as a main course.

8 servings

2 tablespoons olive oil

I large green pepper, cored, seeded, and finely chopped

I large carrot, diced

I medium yellow onion, finely chopped

3 large garlic cloves, chopped

2 tablespoons dried basil

I tablespoon fennel seeds

½ teaspoon crushed dried red pepper flakes

2 quarts chicken stock

2 medium zucchini, cut into ½-inch cubes

4 ounces brown rice, soaked for 30 minutes and drained

3 cups shredded or diced cooked skinless chicken

Salt and freshly ground black pepper

8 teaspoons grated Parmesan cheese

Heat the olive oil in a large heavy saucepan over medium heat. Add the pepper, carrot, onion, and garlic and sauté until the vegetables are tender, about 8 minutes. Meanwhile, crush the basil, fennel seeds, and red pepper flakes together in a spice grinder or with a mortar and pestle. Add to the vegetables and stir.

Pour the broth into the pot. Cover and bring to a boil. Reduce the heat and simmer for 10 minutes. Add the zucchini. Cover and simmer for about 4 minutes, until soft. Raise the heat to high and bring the soup to a boil. Add the rice and boil until tender, about 35 to 40 minutes.

Add the chicken and cook until heated through, 3 to 4 minutes. Season the soup with salt and pepper to taste. Serve in individual bowls and sprinkle each serving with 1 teaspoon Parmesan.

PER SERVING: Calories 237; Fat 13g (Saturated 3g); Cholesterol 34mg; Sodium 1,067mg; Carbohydrates 17g; Fiber 3g (Digestible Carbohydrates 14g); Protein 14g.

Harira

Harira—Moroccan lamb, lentil, and chickpea soup with aromatic spices—is one of my all-time favorite Mediterranean dishes. Even though the legumes put it on the higher end of the spectrum of allowed carbs, I've opted to include it.

8 servings

1 tablespoon unsalted butter

1 tablespoon extra virgin olive oil

1½ pounds boneless lamb shoulder, trimmed and cut into ½-inch cubes

1 large yellow onion, chopped

2 celery stalks, with leaves, chopped

1 teaspoon ground cinnamon

1 teaspoon turmeric

1 teaspoon ground ginger

½ to 1 scant teaspoon cayenne pepper

½ teaspoon saffron threads

2 cups peeled, seeded, and chopped tomatoes, with their juices

Salt

½ cup red lentils, rinsed and picked over

One 14-ounce can chickpeas, drained

½ cup finely chopped flat-leaf parsley

¼ cup finely chopped cilantro

3 to 4 tablespoons fresh lemon juice, to taste

Heat the butter and oil in a large, wide pot over low heat, add the lamb, onion, celery, cinnamon, turmeric, ginger, cayenne, and saffron and cook, stirring, for 8 minutes, until lamb browns lightly.

Add the tomatoes. Raise the heat, bring to a boil, then reduce to a simmer and cook for 15 to 20 minutes, until slightly thickened. Season with salt.

Add the lentils to the pot along with 6 cups water. Bring to a boil, then reduce the heat and simmer, partially covered, for 1½ hours until the lamb is very tender. Add the chickpeas, parsley, and cilantro and cook another 5 to 7 minutes, until the chickpeas are warmed through. Add the lemon juice and serve.

PER SERVING: Calories 226; Fat 9g (Saturated 3g); Cholesterol 53mg; Sodium 319mg; Carbohydrates 17g; Fiber 5g (Digestible Carbohydrates 12g); Protein 20g.

Italian Cabbage-Pork Soup
with Canellini Beans

As I keep mentioning again and again in this book, the limited use of beans and whole grains among the recipes within these pages is my way of tipping my hat to the Mediterranean's fundamental ingredients without losing site of my low-carb intentions. In the Mediterranean, people eat a lot of pulses and legumes, and this hearty winter soup, inspired by one of Marcella Hazan's classic recipes, is sure to soothe souls on cold, blistery days.

8 servings

4 tablespoons extra virgin olive oil

2 ounces lean bacon, cut into $\frac{1}{4}$-inch dice

1 large yellow onion, chopped

2 garlic cloves, chopped

2 medium carrots, diced

2 celery stalks, chopped

1 pound Savoy cabbage, shredded

1 teaspoon dried rosemary

1 scant teaspoon dried thyme

$1\frac{1}{2}$ cup canned chopped Italian plum tomatoes, with their juices

4 cups beef broth

Salt and freshly ground black pepper

4 ounces fresh lean pork sausage

One 14-ounce can canellini beans, drained

Heat 2 tablespoons olive oil and the bacon in a large soup pot over medium heat. When the bacon browns slightly but before it becomes crisp, remove and set aside. Add the onion, garlic, carrot, and celery. Cook until translucent and softened. Add the cabbage, cover, and cook until the cabbage is completely wilted. Add the bacon back to the pot.

Crush the rosemary and thyme together in a spice mill or mortar and pestle and stir into the pot. Add the tomatoes. Bring to a boil, then pour in the broth and 2 cups water. Season with salt and pepper to taste. Reduce the heat and simmer, partially covered, for 1 hour.

Pierce the sausage and brown it in a dry skillet over low heat. Remove from the heat and chop. Add the pork to the soup. In a food processor, puree the remaining olive oil and 3 tablespoons of the beans to a paste and stir into the soup. Add the remaining beans to the soup and simmer another 5 minutes to heat through and serve.

PER SERVING: Calories 169; Fat 9g (Saturated 2g); Cholesterol 8mg; Sodium 698mg; Carbohydrates 14g; Fiber 4g (Digestible Carbohydrates 10g); Protein 8g.

Stracciatella

This light Italian soup makes a perfect starter to one of the hearty vegetable main courses, such as the aromatic cauliflower stew. It's also a lovely to precursor to almost all the chicken recipes in this book.

8 servings

2 quarts chicken broth

2 cups shredded or diced cooked skinless chicken

Salt and freshly ground black pepper

½ cup finely chopped flat-leaf parsley

2 large eggs

½ cup grated Parmesan

½ teaspoon freshly grated nutmeg

2 teaspoons finely grated lemon zest

Place the broth and chicken in a large pot over medium-high heat and bring to a boil. Season with salt and pepper to taste. Add the parsley.

In a medium bowl, vigorously beat together the eggs with the Parmesan, nutmeg, and lemon zest using a fork or small whisk.

Reduce the heat to a simmer. Slowly pour the egg-cheese mixture into the soup, stirring constantly, until the eggs set and form small pieces. Serve immediately.

PER SERVING: Calories 128; Fat 9g (Saturated 3g); Cholesterol 82mg; Sodium 1,275mg; Cabohydrates 1g; Fiber 0g (Digestible Carbohydrates 0g); Protein 11g.

Fish Soups

Andalusian Monkfish Soup with Saffron and Sweet Red Peppers

One could probably write a small book just on the fish soups of the Mediterranean. The Spanish, with their love affair for all foods from the sea, boast some of the best recipes in the region.

8 servings

1 medium potato

5 tablespoons extra virgin olive oil

2 large red peppers, cored, seeded, and diced

2 large garlic cloves, minced

½ teaspoon saffron, crushed to a powder

½ teaspoon ground cumin

½ teaspoon paprika

½ teaspoon cayenne pepper

2 ripe tomatoes, peeled, seeded, and diced

8 cups fish broth

1 pound monkfish or any other firm white-fleshed fish fillets

Salt and freshly ground black pepper

Place the potato in a small pot of salted water over high heat and bring to a boil. When the potato is soft, about 20 minutes, remove from the pot, reserving the potato water. Place the hot potato (do not peel) in a food processor and pulse on and off while drizzling in 1 tablespoon olive oil and 2 tablespoons of the reserved potato water.

Heat 2 tablespoons olive oil in a large soup pot over medium heat. Add the peppers and garlic and sauté for about 1 minute, until just soft. Add the saffron, cumin, paprika, and cayenne and cook, stirring, for 1 minute to release their aroma. Add the tomatoes and their juices, then the potato puree, and stir until smooth.

Pour in the stock. Raise the heat to medium-high and bring to a simmer. Add the fish. Season with salt and pepper to taste. Simmer for 6 to 7 minutes, until the fish is cooked through. Remove from the heat, pour in the remaining 2 tablespoons olive oil, and serve.

PER SERVING: Calories 227; Fat 14g (Saturated 2g); Cholesterol 21mg; Sodium 535mg; Carbohydrates 9g; Fiber 2g (Digestible Carbohydrates 7g); Protein 17g.

Italian Mixed Seafood Soup

This recipe, like many stovetop seafood recipes in Italian cuisine, falls somewhere between soup and stew. Seafood dishes in Italy vary regionally, with the local catch oftentimes determining the recipe. The western, Mediterranean side of Italy provides oily fish, such as sardines, anchovies, and mackerel, which are usually baked with garlic, rosemary, parsley, and any number of other herbs that Italian cooks hold so dear. Shellfish, especially molluscs and crustaceans, come mostly from the Adriatic side of the Boot. The thousands of miles of coast around Italy provide all sorts of other prized catches, too, from hake and shrimp from the Sicilian channel to the oysters and lobsters that go into making Genoa's most famous dish, a pyramid of seafood, eggs, and vegetables called cappon megro. This recipe is one of the easiest to make in the stovetop repertory, a filling soup made with a variety of seafood and a touch of hot pepper. It calls for making a soffrito, which is basically an array of sautéed ingredients such as onions, garlic, and parsley, to which wine and sometimes tomato are added, before the fish or seafood go into the pot. It is a preparation found in many of the seafood and fish soups and stews all around Italy.

8 servings

2 dozen live clams

2 dozen mussels, preferably live, or 24 shelled frozen mussels, defrosted

2 tablespoons extra virgin olive oil

1 large red onion, finely chopped

2 garlic cloves, minced

½ cup chopped flat-leaf parsley

½ cup dry white wine

2 cups chopped fresh peeled, seeded plum tomatoes with their juices,
    or 1½ cups canned plum tomatoes, with their juices

2 pounds cleaned medium squid, cut into ½-inch rings

Salt and freshly ground black pepper

½ teaspoon red pepper flakes

12 medium shrimp, peeled and deveined

12 large sea scallops

Soak the clams in a large pot of cold water, changing the water several times over the course of 2 to 3 hours. Agitate them every so often to loosen the sand from their shells. Drain into a colander and scrub.

If using whole fresh mussels, scrub their shells well and, using a paring knife, cut away their beards.

Heat the olive oil in a large soup pot over medium heat, add the onion and sauté until translucent, about 6 minutes. Add the garlic and cook for about 1 minute, to soften. Stir in the parsley. Pour in the wine and let it sizzle and boil off the alcohol. Add the tomatoes. Reduce the heat, cover the pot, and simmer for 8 minutes, until slightly thickened.

Add the squid to the pot. Cook over low heat, covered, until tender, about 45 minutes. The squid should exude its own liquid. Check the pot occasionally, adding water, if necessary, to keep the squid covered by 1 inch.

Season the soup with salt and pepper to taste and the red pepper flakes. Add the clams and mussels. Cover and raise the heat to medium. As soon as they begin to open, add the shrimp and scallops. Simmer, covered, until the shrimp turns bright pink, the scallops are a glossy white, and the clams and mussels have opened fully. Remove any clams or mussels that haven't opened. Serve immediately.

PER SERVING: Calories 243; Fat 7g (Saturated 1g); Cholesterol 314mg; Sodium 389mg; Carbohydrates 9g; Fiber 1g (Digestible Carbohydrates 8g); Protein 35g.

Greek Sea Bass Soup with
Bulgur and Saffron Avgolemono

There are two main types of fish soups in Greece, those that call for avgolemono, the popular and traditional egg-lemon liaison that thickens so many soups, stews, and sauces, and those that don't. The following soup is a modern interpretation of a Greek classic. Traditionally rice is used to thicken the soup; I have opted for carb-friendlier bulgur wheat. The saffron works very well with the lemon liaison and is a favorite among modern Greek chefs.

8 servings

The Broth

2 large leeks, trimmed and washed well

2 large carrots, trimmed

2 celery stalks, trimmed

2 bay leaves

4 sprigs parsley

4 pounds sea bass, cleaned and gutted but kept whole

Sea salt and freshly ground black pepper

6 tablespoons coarse bulgur

½ teaspoon saffron threads

2 large eggs

Juice of 2 large lemons

⅔ cup olive oil, whisked with the juice of 1 lemon until creamy

Place 2 quarts water in a large soup pot over high heat. Add the leeks, carrots, celery, bay leaves, and parsley and bring to a rolling boil. Reduce the heat, cover partially, and simmer for 45 minutes, skimming the top occasionally. Using a slotted spoon, remove the vegetables and set aside. Remove the bay leaves and parsley and discard.

Place the whole fish in a fine-mesh cheesecloth, tie it tight, and add it to the vegetable broth. Bring to a boil, reduce the heat, and simmer for 35 minutes. Remove the fish and set aside until it is cool enough to handle.

Bring the soup to a boil, season with salt and pepper, and remove ¼ cup. Add the bulgur to the pot and simmer until tender, 10 minutes. Meanwhile, debone the fish and place it on a platter, along with the boiled vegetables, if desired.

Dissolve the saffron in the ¼ cup broth and pour it back into the soup.

In a medium bowl, whisk together the eggs and lemon juice until very frothy. Slowly add a ladleful of the broth, trying to skim it so as not to get any bulgur, into the egg-lemon mixture, whisking all the while. Repeat with another ladleful of soup. Turn off the heat and stir the egg-lemon mixture into the soup. Serve the soup immediately. Drizzle the cleaned fish with the emulsified olive oil–lemon juice mixture, place on a separate platter, and serve along with the soup.

PER SERVING: Calories 252; Fat 20g (Saturated 3g); Cholesterol 63mg; Sodium 200mg; Carbohydrates 12g; Fiber 3g (Digestible Carbohydrates 9g); Protein 8g.

Fruits of the Wine-Dark Sea

ONE OF THE IRONIES OF MEDITERRANEAN FISH COOKERY is that despite the place of honor fish holds in almost all the cuisines, so very few of the traditional dishes translate well in other places. I often hear friends who live in various places around the Mediterranean complaining about the tasteless fish they've sampled across the Atlantic. In Greece, the country I am most familiar with, fish aficionados can pinpoint spots in local waters where they believe the tastiest octopus, or shrimp, or bream or whatever is to be found. It is also difficult to find many of the same species of fish outside the Mediterranean itself.

That said, the recipes that follow are a collection of classic fish and seafood dishes, such as the zarzuela of Spain and the brandade of Provence (in a potato-less, carb-friendly version), as well as recipes that are Mediterranean in spirit, such as the handful of shrimp and mussel recipes at the beginning of the chapter.

Mediterranean fish cookery falls into several broad categories: Simple grilled fish is probably what comes to most people's minds, and, indeed, fresh fish perfectly grilled with a minimum of embellishments is one of the greatest treats the region has to offer. It is not, however, the kind of dish most people are eager to cook at home. In its stead, my paean to whole fish is the recipe for salt-baked fish that my friend and mentor in all things marine, Costas Spiliades, owner of Milos restaurant, shared with me. The Mediterranean is also home to a wealth of other fish dishes beyond the very simplest. There are dozens of great sautéed seafood dishes, and in light of the American love affair with shrimp, I have included several. I also couldn't in good conscience leave out cod, which plays such a central role in Mediterranean fish cookery. Brandade is one example of a classic, king of the classics perhaps. I have included several easy recipes for both salt cod and fresh cod in the form of fillets, both of which are easy to find in American markets.

Monkfish, red snapper, sardines, swordfish, and tuna make up the majority of fish called for in the recipes that follow, although most of the filleted fish dishes may be made with other fish as well, perhaps with easier to find catches, such as perch, halibut, and hake, to name a few.

There are probably as many fish stews in the Mediterranean as there are ports of call, and I wanted to include a few of them here because they are exactly the kind of hearty, rustic fare that gives people far from the wine-dark sea the feeling of coming a little closer to its shores. Moroccan tagines, Sicilian fisherman's stew, the timeless Spanish zarzuela with its variety of fish and seafood are the dishes I chose to include here, nixing a half dozen closer to home (for me) Greek fish stews.

Fish cookery requires a delicate touch, regardless of the recipe. Fresh fish and seafood should never smell either overtly "fishy" or emit even the faintest scent of ammonia. Look a fresh fish in they eye. That's the best advice for detecting exactly how fresh it should be. The eyes should never be dull but should have a deep, tranquil sheen, and the fish itself should be stiff with rigor, not limp. If you must buy frozen, that's fine, too. Much frozen fish, because it is blast-frozen, is oftentimes actually fresher.

Quick and Easy Shrimp and Mussel Dishes

Tarragon-Basil Shrimp

An easy-to-prepare shrimp dish with inarguably French flavors.

2 servings

2 tablespoons unsalted butter
4 shallots, finely chopped
2 garlic cloves, minced
1 pound medium shrimp, peeled and deveined
⅓ cup dry white wine
1 teaspoon dried basil
½ teaspoon dried tarragon
Salt and freshly ground black pepper

Melt the butter in a large nonstick skillet over medium heat. Add the shallots and garlic and sauté for 4 to 5 minutes. Add the shrimp, raise the heat a little, and cook, stirring, until the shrimp turn bright pink, 2 to 3 minutes.

Add the wine, basil, and tarragon. Season with salt and pepper to taste and cook for another 3 to 4 minutes. Remove from the heat and serve.

PER SERVING: Calories 311; Fat 13g (Saturated 8g); Cholesterol 367mg; Sodium 975mg; Carbohydrates 9g; Fiber 1g (Digestible Carbohydrates 8g); Protein 38g.

Shrimp or Mussels in a Skillet with Chardonnay, Fennel, and Feta Sauce

This is a great, easy Greek-inspired shrimp dish that we developed at Pylos for a fall menu.

4 main course servings

---

2 tablespoons extra virgin olive oil, 4 tablespoons if you're using shrimp

1 medium fennel bulb, finely chopped

5 scallions, chopped

1 fresh jalapeño or other chile (or less, to taste), seeded and finely chopped

½ cup dry white wine

24 medium whole shrimp or 40 mussels in the shell, debearded and scrubbed

1 tablespoon fresh lemon juice

4 ounces mild feta, crumbled

Pour 2 tablespoons olive oil into a large, nonreactive skillet over medium-high heat and add the sliced fennel, scallions, and chile. Pour in the wine. Cover the skillet and cook for 7 to 10 minutes, until the sauce is fairly thick. If there isn't enough liquid in the skillet, add up to ½ cup water.

If using shrimp: Heat the remaining 2 tablespoons olive oil in a large, heavy skillet over medium-high heat. Add the shrimp and sauté for about 3 minutes, until they turn bright pink. Empty the shrimp into the skillet with the sauce. Add the lemon juice and feta, reduce the heat to medium, cover, and continue simmering until the cheese melts completely and the sauce is creamy. Serve immediately.

If using mussels: Add the cleaned mussels to the skillet with the sauce. Cover and steam until they open, discarding any that don't. Add the lemon juice and feta, reduce the heat to medium, cover, and continue simmering until the cheese melts completely and the sauce is creamy, 4 to 5 minutes. Serve immediately.

PER SERVING: Calories 260; Fat 20g (Saturated 6g); Cholesterol 80mg; Sodium 403mg; Carbohydrates 8g; Fiber 2g (Digestible Carbohydrates 6g); Protein 12g.

Pan-Seared Shrimp with Romesco Sauce

Romesco sauce is a pungent, garlicky Catalan pepper sauce traditionally served with grilled fish and seafood.

6 servings

The Romesco

1 tablespoon extra virgin olive oil

½ cup chopped yellow onion

3 garlic cloves, minced

1 roasted red pepper in brine, drained and chopped

1 fresh chile, roasted, peeled, seeded, and chopped

2 medium ripe tomatoes, peeled, seeded, and chopped, with their juices

¾ cup fish stock or clam juice

¼ cup dry white wine

¼ cup blanched almonds

¼ cup hazelnuts

2 tablespoons sherry or red wine vinegar

Salt and freshly ground black pepper

The shrimp

1 tablespoon olive oil

24 large shrimp, peeled and deveined, with heads left on

Sea salt

1 lemon, cut into 4 to 6 wedges

Prepare the sauce: Heat the olive oil in a large, heavy skillet over medium heat, add the onions, and sauté for 5 minutes, until softened. Add the garlic, roasted red pepper, and chile and stir. Add the tomatoes. Cook for about 5 minutes, until some of the juices boil off. Add the stock and wine. Cover, reduce the heat to a simmer, and cook for 30 minutes.

Meanwhile, lightly toast the almonds and hazelnuts in a dry skillet over low heat. Remove from the heat, cool slightly, and grind in a food processor until mealy and granular. Add the vinegar and pulse to combine. Remove the tomato mixture from the heat, let it cool for a few minutes, and add it to the nut mixture in the food processor. Pulse to blend. Add salt and pepper to taste and set the sauce aside.

Heat a heavy nonstick skillet or ribbed stovetop griddle over medium-high heat. If using a skillet, add 1 tablespoon olive oil and tilt the pan to coat it. If using a griddle, brush the surface with 1 tablespoon olive oil. Raise the heat to high, place the shrimp in the skillet or griddle, and sear until they turn bright pink, about 4 minutes. Flip and sear on the other side. Season with salt and serve hot with the Romesco sauce and lemon wedges on the side.

PER SERVING: Calories, 165; Fat 12g (Saturated 1g); Cholesterol 43mg; Sodium 395mg; Carbohydrates 9g; Fiber 3g (Digestible Carbohydrates 6g); Protein 8g.

Sautéed Shrimp Served with Saffron Avgolemono and Seared Zucchini

Another simple shrimp dish from Pylos, a Greek restaurant on East 7th Street in New York City, where I am consulting chef.

4 servings

3 cups vegetable broth

16 medium shrimp, peeled and deveined (reserve the shells for broth)

½ teaspoon saffron, crushed and dissolved in 2 tablespoons warm water

1 egg

Juice of 1 lemon

2 tablespoons extra virgin olive oil

1 large garlic clove, smashed

4 medium zucchini, trimmed and quartered lengthwise

Salt and freshly ground black pepper

1 garlic clove, thinly sliced

½ cup dry white wine

Make the sauce: Place the broth and shrimp shells in a medium pot over high heat. Bring to a boil and boil for about 30 minutes, or until reduced to 1 cup. Strain, reserving the broth. Add the saffron to the hot broth and stir. In a small bowl, whisk together the egg and lemon juice. Place the broth back on the stove, bring to a gentle simmer, and add a small ladleful of the broth to the egg-lemon mixture, whisking all the while. Add another small ladleful, whisking. Pour the egg-lemon mixture into the pot, turn off the heat, and swirl to combine. Set aside.

Heat 1 tablespoon olive oil with the smashed garlic in a large nonstick skillet. As soon as the garlic begins to color, remove it. Add the zucchini and sauté over high heat for 5 to 6 minutes, until tender but still firm. Season with salt and pepper to taste and remove from the skillet. Cover to keep warm.

In the same skillet, heat the remaining tablespoon olive oil over medium heat. Add the shrimp and sliced garlic and sauté for 2 to 3 minutes, until the shrimp turn pink. Add the wine and raise the heat to steam off the alcohol. Reduce the heat, add the egg-lemon mixture to the skillet, and stir gently to thicken slightly. Remove from the heat. Place the zucchini on a platter or on individual plates and serve the shrimp and sauce over it. Serve immediately.

PER SERVING: Calories 154; Fat 10g (Saturated 1g); Cholesterol 90mg; Sodium 1,389mg; Carbohydrates 10g; Fiber 3g (Digestible Carbohydrates 7g); Protein 10g.

The Simplest Pan-Mediterranean Shrimp

Shrimp sautéed with the trio of pan-Mediterranean flavors: garlic, lemon, and herbs.

4 servings

---

4 tablespoons extra virgin olive oil

3 tablespoons fresh lemon juice

4 tablespoons dry white wine

3 garlic cloves, minced

1½ pounds medium shrimp, peeled and deveined

½ teaspoon dried marjoram

½ teaspoon crushed red pepper flakes

Salt

3 tablespoons chopped flat-leaf parsley

Whisk together 3 tablespoons olive oil, the lemon juice, wine, and garlic in a medium bowl. Toss in the shrimp. Cover and let stand in the refrigerator for 20 to 30 minutes.

Heat the remaining tablespoon olive oil in a large nonstick skillet over high heat. Remove the shrimp from the marinade with a slotted spoon and add to the skillet. Cook for about 3 minutes, stirring, until the shrimp become bright pink. Remove the shrimp from the skillet to a serving platter. Add the marinade, marjoram, and red pepper flakes to the skillet. Reduce the heat to medium and simmer for about 5 minutes.

Return the shrimp back to the skillet, heat through, season with salt to taste, and toss with the parsley. Serve immediately.

PER SERVING: Calories 228; Fat 12g (Saturated 2g); Cholesterol 252mg; Sodium 583mg; Carbohydrates 2g; Fiber 0g (Digestible Carbohydrates 2g); Protein 27g.

Garlicky Sautéed Shrimp

A few years ago I met up with some friends in Spain for an unruly three days of tapas bar–hopping. I based this dish on one we had at a small tapas bar in Barcelona.

4 servings

3 tablespoons extra virgin olive oil

2 red peppers, cored, seeded, and cut into ½-inch strips

2 green peppers, cored, seeded, and cut into ½-inch strips

4 large garlic cloves, slivered

2 ounces Spanish ham such as serrano, chopped

¼ to ½ teaspoon cayenne pepper

1½ pounds medium shrimp, peeled and deveined

½ cup dry sherry

Salt and freshly ground black pepper

3 tablespoons chopped flat-leaf parsley

Heat 2 tablespoons olive oil in a large nonstick skillet over medium heat, add the peppers and sauté until wilted, 6 to 7 minutes. Add the garlic and cook, stirring, for 1 minute. Add the ham and cayenne and cook for about 1 minute.

Heat the remaining olive oil in a separate large nonstick skillet over high heat, add the shrimp, and sear it, turning once, until bright pink, about 2 minutes.

Transfer the shrimp and their juices to the skillet with the peppers. Raise the heat to high and add the sherry. As soon as it steams up, reduce the heat. Season with salt and pepper to taste and cook for about 2 minutes, until the flavors meld. Remove from the heat, sprinkle with the parsley, and serve.

PER SERVING: Calories 288; Fat 14g (Saturated 2g); Cholesterol 264mg; Sodium 858mg; Carbohydrates 9g; Fiber 3g (Digestible Carbohydrates 6g); Protein 32g.

Shrimp and Mussels in a
Summertime Tomato Sauce

On the island of Ikaria, where we spend our summers, the garden is fragrant with several varieties of basil and mounds of my husband's organic tomatoes. It is important to use good, preferably organic, tomatoes for this and many other dishes in this book. It's also important to save this dish for summer, when tomatoes are in season.

6 servings

6 ripe tomatoes

4 tablespoons extra virgin olive oil

I small red onion, minced

3 garlic cloves, smashed

Salt and freshly ground black pepper

I cup chopped mixed varieties of fresh basil (Italian basil, cinnamon basil,
   purple basil, tiny-leaved basil)

½ cup chopped fresh oregano

I½ pounds medium shrimp, peeled and deveined

⅔ cup dry white wine

24 mussels, scrubbed and debearded

Chop 3 tomatoes and puree the remaining 3 in a food processor. Heat 2 tablespoons of the olive oil in a large, wide, shallow pot or deep skillet over medium heat, add the onion and garlic, and sauté for about 5 minutes, until soft. Add the chopped tomatoes and pureed tomatoes. Season with salt and pepper to taste. Reduce the heat to low, partially cover the pot, and simmer for about 40–45 minutes, until thick. Add the basil and oregano and cook another 5 to 10 minutes, then remove from the heat.

During the last 10 minutes of cooking, heat the remaining 2 tablespoons olive oil in a large nonstick skillet over high heat, add the shrimp, and sauté for 3 to 4 minutes, until they turn bright pink. Place the wine and mussels in a large nonreactive pot over high heat. Cover the pot, bring to a boil, and steam for 6 to 7 minutes, until the mussels open, discarding any that don't. Drain the mussels and add them, along with the shrimp, to the tomato sauce. Cover and cook for about 5 minutes, until the flavors meld, and serve.

PER SERVING: Calories 283; Fat 13g (Saturated 2g); Cholesterol 191mg; Sodium 631mg; Carbohydrates 13g; Fiber 2g (Digestible Carbohydrates 11g); Protein 30g.

Spicy Steamed Spanish-Style Mussels

I found this recipe in a pamphlet about seafood in the Mediterranean, liked the sound of it, and adapted it.

8 servings

80 mussels, scrubbed and debearded

2 cups dry white wine

¾ cup blanched almonds

½ cup pine nuts

4 garlic cloves, chopped

½ cup chopped flat-leaf parsley

3 tablespoons extra virgin olive oil

1 large onion, very finely chopped

2 teaspoons paprika

½ to 1 teaspoon cayenne pepper

1½ cups chopped plum tomatoes, with their juices

2 teaspoons tomato paste

Salt

Place the mussels in a large pot along with 2 cups water and the wine. Place over high heat, cover, and steam for 6 to 7 minutes, until the mussels open, discarding any that don't. Remove the mussels with a slotted spoon to a bowl, strain the pot juices, and set aside.

Place the almonds, pine nuts, garlic, parsley, and 1 tablespoon olive oil in a food processor and puree to a paste.

Heat the remaining 2 tablespoons olive oil in a large nonstick skillet over medium heat, add the onion and cook, until wilted, about 5 minutes. Add the paprika, cayenne, tomatoes, and tomato paste. Add the nut mixture and enough of the pot juices from the mussels to make a very thick sauce. Add salt to taste.

Arrange the mussels on a serving platter and spoon a little of the sauce into each of them. Serve immediately.

PER SERVING: Calories 334; Fat 20g (Saturated 3g); Cholesterol 45mg; Sodium 617mg; Carbohydrates 14g; Fiber 3g (Digestible Carbohydrates 11g); Protein 25g.

Brandade in Romaine Lettuce Leaves
with Roasted Red Peppers

Brandade is the famed Provençal salt cod cream, one of the standard bearers of Mediter-ranean cuisine. Usually served with aioli, with potatoes, or on bread, I serve it here in crisp endive leaves, topped with the sweet touch of roasted red peppers. Remember that salt cod must be soaked in several changes of water over a forty-eight hour period, so plan ahead.

8 servings

---

1 pound salt cod fillet

7 tablespoons extra virgin olive oil

4 tablespoons finely chopped onion

2 garlic cloves, finely chopped

3 tablespoons light cream

1 to 2 tablespoons fresh lemon juice, to taste

Salt and freshly ground black pepper

2 red peppers, roasted, peeled, cored, and seeded

8 crisp romaine leaves

1 lemon, cut into thin rounds, for garnish

Soak the cod in a shallow dish of cold water in the refrigerator, changing the water 3 to 4 times over the course of 48 hours.

Bring a large pot of water to a boil and blanch the cod for 10 to 15 minutes, until flaky and cooked through. Remove, pat dry, and flake, removing any bones.

Heat 2 tablespoons olive oil in a small skillet over medium heat, add the onion and garlic and cook, stirring, until translucent, 5 to 7 minutes.

Place the cod and onion-garlic mixture in a food processor. While the processor is run-ning, slowly add 4 tablespoons olive oil, the cream, and lemon juice in alternating streams, until the mixture is the consistency of a mousse. Season with salt and pepper to taste, if desired. Remove the mixture to a bowl.

Wipe or rinse the food processor bowl clean and process the peppers and the remaining tablespoon olive oil for a few seconds until coarsely pureed.

Trim the tough bottom ends off the lettuce leaves. Place 2 heaping tablespoons of the cod mixture in each lettuce leaf and top with a dollop of the pepper mixture. Garnish with the lemon rounds and serve.

PER SERVING: Calories 302; Fat 14g (Saturated 3g); Cholesterol 90mg; Sodium 560mg; Carbohydrates 5g; Fiber 3g (Digestible Carbohydrates 2g); Protein 37g.

Spicy Basque-Style Salt Cod

The Basque, whose fishing boats made it to the shores of the Americas long before Columbus's did, were the most renowned cod fishermen in the world. They developed the technique for preserving cod in salt, which in turn became salvation at sea for generations of sailors. It was by following the Basque that the Vikings learned of the great schools of cod off the coast of New England. For centuries, salt cod was the landlubber's fish throughout the Mediterranean, hawked by itinerant merchants who transported the preserved fish into the remotest villages. For centuries, too, cod was a poor man's fish, entrenched in almost all the cooking traditions of the region. That has changed nowadays, as schools of cod are in ever-short supply, yet it remains one of the mainstays of the Mediterranean table.

4 servings

I pound salt cod fillet

¼ cup extra virgin olive oil

I cup chopped yellow onion

4 red peppers, cored, seeded, and chopped

2 garlic cloves, chopped

2 large hard-boiled egg yolks

3 tablespoons chopped flat-leaf parsley

2 small hot dry chiles or ½ to I scant teaspoon cayenne pepper, to taste

¼ cup dry white wine

I cup clam juice or water

Soak the cod in a shallow dish of cold water, in the refrigerator, changing the water 3 to 4 times over the course of 48 hours. Once soaked, drain and cut the cod into 4 pieces.

Preheat the oven to 350°F.

Heat I tablespoon olive oil in a nonstick ovenproof skillet over medium heat, add the onions, peppers, and garlic, and sauté for about 5 minutes.

Crumble the egg yolks into the mixture, reduce the heat, cover, and cook for 3 to 4 more minutes, until soft. Transfer the mixture to a food processor, add the parsley and chile and pulse to puree. Return the mixture to the skillet, heat over medium heat, and add the wine. As soon as the wine evaporates, add the clam juice or water. Cover and simmer for 10 minutes.

Place the cod in the skillet and spoon the sauce over the fish evenly to cover. Drizzle the remaining 3 tablespoons olive oil over the fish. Bake, uncovered, for 25 minutes, or until the fish is fork tender and flaky. Serve immediately.

PER SERVING: Calories 540; Fat 20g (Saturated 3g); Cholesterol 279mg; Sodium 872mg; Carbohydrates 12g; Fiber 3g (Digestible Carbohydrates 9g); Protein 76g.

Basque-Style Salt Cod with Red Peppers, Onions, and Herbs

Cod and peppers are a frequent combination in the hearty cookery of the Basque. Also common in the cooking from that part of the Mediterranean, as witnessed in the previous recipe and many others not in this book, is the addition of hard-boiled eggs to various fish dishes. The egg, in fact, offsets some of the residual saltiness of the cod and adds another layer of texture.

4 servings

1 pound salt cod fillet

2 tablespoons diced lean bacon

½ cup trimmed, diced Spanish ham, such as Serrano

1 tablespoon extra virgin olive oil

1½ cups finely chopped onion

2 garlic cloves, minced

2 tablespoons chopped flat-leaf parsley

⅔ cup chopped roasted red peppers

1 large hard-boiled egg yolk, crumbled

1 bay leaf

½ teaspoon hot paprika or cayenne pepper

½ cup dry white wine

Start this dish 2 days beforehand by soaking the cod: Place the cod in a large pot filled with cold water and let it soak in the refrigerator for 48 hours, changing the water at least 4 times. Drain and cut the cod into serving portions.

Place the bacon in a large, deep skillet or wide, shallow pot over low heat and cook until golden but not tough. Add the ham and cook, stirring, for about 3 minutes, until lightly browned. Remove the bacon and ham from the skillet and set aside. Drain off some of the fat, leaving about 1 tablespoon in the skillet for flavor. Add the olive oil, raise the heat to medium, add the onion and garlic, and cook until wilted, about 5 minutes. Add the parsley, reduce the heat to low, and cook, covered, until the onion is very soft but not browned, about 15 minutes.

Add the roasted red peppers to the onion mixture. Then add the crumbled egg yolk and the bacon-ham mixture to the skillet. Next, add the bay leaf, paprika, wine, and ½ cup water. Raise heat and boil off the alcohol for about 1 minute.

Remove half the mixture with a slotted spoon and set aside. Reduce the heat to medium and spread the remaining mixture evenly over the surface of the skillet. Place the cod on top and cover with the other half of the onion-pepper mixture. Cover and cook until the fish is fork tender, about 12 minutes. Remove carefully and serve.

PER SERVING: Calories 437; Fat 8g (Saturated 2g); Cholesterol 184mg; Sodium 1,407mg; Carbohydrates 10g; Fiber 1g (Digestible Carbohydrates 9g); Protein 77g.

Cod Fillets with Orange and Cracked Green Olive Salsa

Oranges and olives are the telltale signs of the cooking of Morocco, whence this fresh cod dish originally hails.

4 servings

The Salsa

1 small navel orange

4 fresh plum tomatoes, peeled, seeded, and chopped

2 tablespoons fresh orange juice

⅓ cup finely chopped red onion

2 tablespoons fresh strained lemon juice

2 tablespoons extra virgin olive oil

½ cup finely chopped pitted Greek cracked green olives

½ teaspoon crushed coriander seeds

½ teaspoon smoked Hungarian paprika or sweet paprika

1 tablespoon capers, drained and finely chopped

2 teaspoons fresh marjoram or oregano

The Fish

Four 6-ounce cod or other white-fleshed fish fillets such as halibut or perch

Salt and freshly ground black pepper

2 teaspoons finely chopped lemon zest

2 teaspoons finely chopped orange zest

2 tablespoons extra virgin olive oil

Make the salsa: Scrape the orange against the fine-toothed side of a hand grater and save the zest for the fish. Peel the orange, removing the pith completely. Cut the orange into

¼-inch dice. Combine all the salsa ingredients in a bowl, cover, and let stand for 1 hour, refrigerated. Remove from the refrigerator 15 to 20 minutes before serving.

Preheat the oven to 375°F. Lightly oil a glass ovenproof baking dish large enough to fit the fish in 1 layer. Season the fish on both sides with salt and pepper to taste. Place in the pan and sprinkle with the orange and lemon zests. Drizzle with the olive oil. Bake for about 12 minutes, until the fish is fork tender. Remove to a platter, spoon over the salsa and any pan juices, and serve.

PER SERVING: Calories 320; Fat 18g (Saturated 2g); Cholesterol 65mg; Sodium 1,015mg; Carbohydrates 13g; Fiber 2g (Digestible Carbohydrates 11g); Protein 28g.

Whole Baked Fish

Whole Fish with Herbs in a Salt Crust

My friend and fish master Costas Spiliades, chef-owner of Milos restaurants in Montreal, New York, and Athens, helped me perfect this dish. His Milos Athens restaurant serves this. Salt-crusted fish is easy to do at home and makes a dramatic presentation.

4 servings

One 2½- to 3-pound whole fish, such as sea bass, grouper, or sea bream, cleaned and
  gutted, but not scaled
2 celery stalks, coarsely chopped
1 small fennel bulb, coarsely chopped
2 to 3 thyme sprigs
2 to 3 parsley sprigs
4 pounds kosher salt
¼ cup olive oil
2 to 3 tablespoons fresh lemon juice
Salt and freshly ground black pepper

Preheat the oven to 450°F.

Fill the cavity of the fish with the celery, fennel, thyme, and parsley.

Place the salt in a large basin and mix with 1 cup water. The mixture will become dense and will have enough moisture to adhere naturally to the fish. You may need a little more water to achieve this. Spread a layer of the salt mixture on the bottom of a baking dish large enough to hold the fish with room to spare and without bending it. Place the fish on top of the salt and add the remaining salt to the pan, covering the fish completely and mounding it all around. You can leave a part of the head exposed near the cheek, if desired, to make testing for doneness easier.

Bake the fish, uncovered, for 20 to 25 minutes (the general rule is 10 to 12 minutes per pound).

While the fish is baking, whisk together the olive oil and lemon juice in a small bowl and season lightly with salt and pepper.

Remove the fish from the oven. Using a sharp knife, crack open the salt and dislodge it from the fish. Place the fish on a serving platter and serve with the dressing on the side.

PER SERVING: Calories 255; Fat 15g (Saturated 2g); Cholesterol 53mg; Sodium 351mg; Carbohydrates 1g; Fiber 0g (Digestible Carbohydrates 1g); Protein 28g.

Braised Sardines in Grape Leaves

This dish takes its cue from a classic Spanish dish, Santander Style, in which the sardines are wrapped in grape leaves and poached. Greeks make sardines wrapped in grape leaves, too, but they generally either grill or bake the fish. I have taken liberties with the traditions from both ends of the Mediterranean. Fresh sardines braised in the oven instead of on the stovetop tend to hold together rather than fall apart.

4 servings

12 brine-preserved grape leaves

12 medium sardines, gutted

2 tablespoons extra virgin olive oil

3 scallions, upper greens trimmed, finely chopped

2 garlic cloves, minced

4 medium ripe tomatoes, seeded and chopped

⅓ cup dry white wine

¼ cup chopped flat-leaf parsley

¼ cup chopped fresh mint

Salt and freshly ground black pepper

½ teaspoon paprika

Blanch the grape leaves in a pot of boiling water for 3 minutes. Remove with a slotted spoon to a colander and rinse under cold water.

Lightly oil an ovenproof glass baking dish large enough to hold the sardines snuggly in 1 layer. Preheat the oven to 350°F.

Heat 1 tablespoon olive oil in a medium skillet over medium heat, add the scallions and garlic, and cook until soft, about 5 minutes. Add the tomatoes and wine and cook, uncovered, for 5 to 7 minutes, just until the tomatoes begin to loose some of their water. Toss in the parsley and mint and remove from the heat.

Season each sardine with salt and pepper to taste and wrap each in a grape leaf. Place seam side down in the baking dish. Distribute the sauce evenly over the sardines. Drizzle in the remaining 6 tablespoons olive oil. Sprinkle with the paprika. Cover the pan with foil and bake for about 35 minutes, until the fish is flaky and tender. Remove from the oven and place 3 sardines on each plate, with the sauce spooned on top.

PER SERVING: Calories 245; Fat 15g (Saturated 3g); Cholesterol 52mg; Sodium 1,057mg; Carbohydrates 10g; Fiber 2g (Digestible Carbohydrates 8g); Protein 18g.

Red Mullet Baked in Parchment Paper

Red mullet, rouget *to the French,* triglia *to the Italians,* salmonete *to the Spanish,* mellou *to the Tunisians, is a quintessentially Mediterranean fish. Since it is not readily available in North American fish markets, substitute any small, whole firm-fleshed, delicate-flavored fish, such as porgies. Salmon steaks also work well; bake for 15 minutes.*

4 servings

4 whole red mullets (8 ounces each), scaled and gutted

Salt and freshly ground black pepper

4 tablespoons olive oil

1 tablespoon fresh lemon juice

2 tablespoons ouzo or other anise-flavored liqueur

1 medium red onion, cut into 12 thin rounds

1 medium ripe tomato, cut into 8 rounds

4 teaspoons small capers, drained

4 tablespoons chopped flat-leaf parsley

1 lemon, sliced into 8 rounds

Season the fish inside and out with salt and pepper to taste. Whisk together the olive oil, lemon juice, and ouzo in a large bowl, add the fish and coat with the marinade. Cover and marinate in the refrigerator for 1 hour.

Preheat the oven to 350°F. Remove the fish from the marinade, reserving it. Place 1 fish on one of four 8-inch square pieces of parchment paper. Top the fish with 3 onion slices, covering the body of the fish as much as possible, followed by 2 tomato slices, then 1 teaspoon capers, 1 tablespoon parsley, and 2 lemon rounds. Drizzle the fish with a little of the marinade. Fold the paper over the fish to make a secure parcel, turning the top edges in together to seal. Repeat with the other 3 fish.

Lightly oil a baking dish large enough to hold all the parcels. Place the parcels seam side up in the pan and sprinkle with a little water. Bake for about 30 minutes, until the fish is tender. Serve on individual plates, each fish in its parcel.

PER SERVING: Calories 312; Fat 19g (Saturated 4g); Cholesterol 71mg; Sodium 463mg; Carbohydrates 5g; Fiber 1g (Digestible Carbohydrates 4g); Protein 29g.

Red Snapper with Almond, Paprika, and Herb Sauce

4 servings

1 small head garlic
½ cup chopped flat-leaf parsley
¼ cup chopped fresh oregano
¼ cup chopped fresh mint
½ cup ground blanched almonds
2 teaspoons paprika
3 tablespoons extra virgin olive oil
2 cups hot fish or vegetable stock
Four 8-ounce red snapper, striped bass, or other firm white-fleshed fillets

Using a mortar and pestle or a food processor, pulverize the garlic, parsley, oregano, mint, almonds, paprika, and 1 tablespoon olive oil to a paste.

Heat the remaining 2 tablespoons olive oil in a large, heavy skillet over medium heat and add the paste. Cook for 1 to 2 minutes, stirring, to release the aromas of the nuts and herbs. Slowly add the hot broth, stirring. After all the broth has been added, raise the heat, bring to a boil, then reduce the heat to low and cook, stirring, until the mixture thickens, 10 to 12 minutes.

While the sauce is simmering, preheat the oven to 350°F and lightly oil a shallow baking dish large enough to hold the fish in 1 layer. Place the fish on the bottom of the dish, cover evenly with the sauce, and bake for about 12 minutes, until the fish is flaky. Serve immediately.

PER SERVING: Calories 415; Fat 20g (Saturated 3g); Cholesterol 81 mg; Sodium 289mg; Carbohydrates 6g; Fiber 2g (Digestible Carbohydrates 4g); Protein 51g.

Sautéed Monkfish with Pine Nuts, Saffron, and Tomatoes

Monkfish is arguably one of the most unattractive fish in the sea, all head and tail with seemingly nothing in between. Yet for all its ungainliness, it is one of the most delicious fish.

4 servings

3 tablespoons extra virgin olive oil

²⁄₃ cup chopped onion

1 garlic clove, chopped

2 tablespoons pine nuts

2 ripe tomatoes, peeled, seeded, and finely chopped, with their juices,
    or 1 cup canned chopped plum tomatoes, with their juices

¼ teaspoon saffron threads, crushed in a mortar

1½ pounds monkfish or other firm-fleshed delicately flavored fish fillets,
    cut into 2-inch strips

Salt and freshly ground black pepper

Heat 1 tablespoon olive oil in a medium nonstick skillet over medium heat, add the onion and garlic, and sauté for 5 minutes, until soft. Add the pine nuts and cook, stirring, for 2 to 3 more minutes. Add the tomatoes and bring to a simmer. Cook, stirring, for 6 to 7 minutes, until the sauce begins to thicken.

Add the saffron and stir to combine. Remove the pan from the heat and set aside.

Heat the remaining 2 tablespoons olive oil in a separate large nonstick skillet over medium-high heat. Season the monkfish with salt and pepper to taste and sauté for 1 minute on each side. Pour the sauce into the skillet, reduce the heat, and cook for another 8 to 10 minutes, until the fish is flaky. Remove from the heat and serve.

PER SERVING: Calories 265; Fat 15g (Saturated 2g); Cholesterol 41 mg; Sodium 328mg; Carbohydrates 7g; Fiber 2g (Digestible Carbohydrates 5g); Protein 26g.

Monkfish Sautéed with Portobello Mushrooms, Shallots, and Herbs

Here's another easy recipe for one of the sea's most flavourful bounties, inspired by classic French cooking.

4 servings

1½ pounds monkfish fillets

Salt and freshly ground black pepper

1 tablespoon extra virgin olive oil

2 tablespoons unsalted butter

4 shallots, thinly sliced

1 large garlic clove, minced

½ pound portobello mushrooms, trimmed and cut into 1-inch strips

⅓ cup dry white wine

3 tablespoons finely chopped flat-leaf parsley

1 teaspoon dried tarragon

Season the monkfish with salt and pepper and set aside until ready to use.

Heat the butter in a large nonstick skillet over medium heat. Add the shallots and garlic and sauté for 1 minute. Add the mushrooms, season with salt and pepper to taste, reduce the heat, cover, and cook for about 8 minutes, until tender.

Heat the olive oil in a separate nonstick skillet over high heat, add the fish, and sauté for about 2 minutes per side, until opaque. Remove and cut into 1-inch strips.

Raise the heat under the mushrooms and add the wine. When it steams up, in just a few seconds, lower the heat and toss in the parsley, tarragon, and remaining tablespoon butter. Raise the heat to high and stir with a wooden spoon for about 3 to 4 minutes until wilted. Add the fish to the mushrooms. Reduce the heat to medium, cover, and cook to warm through, about 3 minutes. Remove from the heat, season with additional salt and pepper, if desired, and serve.

PER SERVING: Calories 177; Fat 8g (Saturated 3g); Cholesterol 35mg; Sodium 319mg; Carbohydrates 6g; Fiber 1g (Digestible Carbohydrates 5g); Protein 17g.

Tuna alla Livornese

Tuna has been of immense importance to the Mediterranean since time immemorial. The late food historian Alan Davidson wrote that tuna traps may have been set as long ago as Neolithic times. Today, tuna fishing remains an important part of the Mediterranean fisherman's livelihood, even though the prized blue fin as well as other species are in dwindling supply. Tuna is a fish that raises eyebrows for many reasons these days, first because of its ever-decreasing numbers but also for the fact that, like many other fatty fish, it tends to be a magnet for all the ocean's ills, especially mercury. It is a delicious fish; it just needs to be eaten judiciously. But then, what doesn't?

6 servings

The Sauce

1 tablespoon extra virgin olive oil

1 cup chopped red onion

4 garlic cloves, minced

6 medium ripe tomatoes, finely chopped, with their juices

⅓ cup chopped flat-leaf parsley

⅓ cup chopped fresh basil

½ cup dry white wine

24 Kalamata olives, pitted and chopped

2 tablespoons capers, rinsed and chopped

The Fish

2 tablespoons olive oil

Six 6-ounce tuna steaks, about 1 inch thick

Salt and freshly ground black pepper

Prepare the sauce: Heat the extra virgin olive oil in a large, wide, shallow pot or deep skillet, add the onion and cook, stirring, until soft and translucent, about 8 minutes.

Add the garlic and stir once or twice. Add the tomatoes, parsley, and basil and cook until the sauce begins to thicken, about 15 minutes.

While the sauce is cooking, heat 1 tablespoon olive oil in a separate large skillet over high heat and sear the tuna, 3 steaks at a time, if they fit into the pan, for 2 minutes on each side, until lightly charred. Season with salt and pepper to taste just before removing. Repeat with the remaining 3 steaks.

Toss the olives and capers into the sauce and mix. Add the fish. Cover and cook for 3 to 4 minutes, until cooked through and medium-rare. Do not overcook the tuna. Remove from the heat and serve.

PER SERVING: Calories 315; Fat 13g (Saturated 2g); Cholesterol 69mg; Sodium 595mg; Carbohydrates 12g; Fiber 3g (Digestible Carbohydrates 9g); Protein 38g.

Tuna Steak Stimpereta

Here is my adaption of Marcella Hazan's recipe in Essentials of Classic Italian Cooking.

4 servings

3 tablespoons extra virgin olive oil

Four 6-ounce tuna or other firm-fleshed fish fillets, about ¾ inch thick

Salt and freshly ground black pepper

½ cup very finely chopped red onion

¾ cup finely chopped celery

2 tablespoons small capers in brine, drained

2 tablespoons golden raisins, plumped in 3 tablespoons warm water

¼ cup white wine vinegar

Heat I tablespoon olive oil in a large nonstick skillet over medium-high heat. Sauté 2 fillets for about 3 minutes, until lightly seared or opaque. Season lightly with salt and pepper, turn carefully, and cook another 2 to 3 minutes, until the fish is fork tender. Season the other side with salt and pepper just before removing from the skillet. Remove from the skillet, add another tablespoon olive oil, and cook the other two fillets in the same manner. Cover and set aside.

Heat the remaining oil in the same skillet over medium heat. Add the onion and celery and cook until translucent, about 5 minutes. Add the capers and raisins and their water. Simmer until the water cooks off, about 3 minutes. Place the fish over the mixture and pour in the vinegar. Cover and cook for about 3 to 4 minutes, until fish is fork tender. Season with salt and pepper to taste and serve.

PER SERVING: Calories 296; Fat 12g (Saturated 2g); Cholesterol 74mg; Sodium 501mg; Carbohydrates 7g; Fiber Ig (Digestible Carbohydrates 6g); Protein 39g.

A Few Fish Stews

Sicilian Fisherman's Stew

Fish stews abound throughout the Mediterranean and most evolved from the fishing boats themselves, as fishermen reserved the worst of their catch for themselves and cooked it on-board. The following two recipes are two of my personal favorites from the Mediterranean repertoire.

4 servings

2 tablespoons extra virgin olive oil

1 cup chopped red onion

2 garlic cloves, chopped

1 cup finely chopped flat-leaf parsley

2 medium ripe tomatoes, peeled, seeded, and finely chopped, with their juices

½ cup dry white wine

2 pounds mixed fresh fish fillets such as snapper, cod, sea bass, swordfish, tile fish, and halibut, cut into large pieces

Salt and freshly ground black pepper

Heat the olive oil in a wide, heavy pot over medium heat, add the onions and garlic, and cook, stirring occasionally, until translucent, about 5 minutes. Add the parsley and tomatoes. Raise the heat and bring to a simmer. Add 1 cup water and the wine.

Cook, partially covered, for 10 minutes. Add the fish, cover, and simmer for 12 to 15 minutes. Season with salt and pepper to taste and serve.

PER SERVING: Calories 318; Fat 10g (Saturated 2g); Cholesterol 80mg; Sodium 404mg; Carbohydrates 9g; Fiber 2g (Digestible Carbohydrates 7g); Protein 46g.

Zarzuela

Some versions of this seafood potpourri, named after the light satirical operas that were im-mensely popular in nineteenth century Spain, contain both fish and shellfish; others contain bread and nuts; and some are spiced with chiles.

6 servings

2 tablespoons extra virgin olive oil

¾ cup finely chopped yellow onion

2 garlic cloves, minced

I pound fresh squid, cleaned and cut into ½-inch rings, tentacles chopped

Salt and freshly ground black pepper

2 tablespoons brandy

2 ripe tomatoes, peeled, seeded, and finely chopped

I teaspoon paprika

½ teaspoon cayenne pepper

¼ teaspoon saffron threads, crumbled

2 bay leaves

½ cup dry white wine

2 cups fish stock or clam juice

½ pound sea bass, cod, hake, or halibut fillets, cut into I-inch strips

½ pound monkfish fillets, cut into I-inch strips

18 mussels, scrubbed and debearded

18 clams, scrubbed

I pound large shrimp, peeled and deveined

4 tablespoons chopped flat-leaf parsley

Heat the olive oil in a large, wide pot or Dutch oven over medium heat, add the onions, and cook until tender, about 6 to 7 minutes. Add the garlic and continue cooking, stir-ring, for about 2 minutes. Add the squid, season with salt and pepper to taste, and cook for 1 minute, until the squid turns opaque. Add the brandy. When the alcohol cooks off, in about 2 to 3 minutes, add the tomatoes, paprika, cayenne, saffron, and bay leaves. Raise the heat to high and bring to a boil. Add the wine. When the wine steams off, add the clam juice, bring to a boil, reduce heat to low, partially cover the pot, and simmer for 15 to 20 minutes, until thick.

Add the fish fillets, mussels, clams, and shrimp to the pot. Season with salt and pepper to taste. Cover and cook until the mussels and clams open, about 10 minutes. Remove and discard any mussels or clams that have not opened. Add the parsley and tilt the pot back and forth to distribute it. Remove the pan from the heat and serve.

PER SERVING: Calories 306; Fat 9g (Saturated 2g); Cholesterol 334mg; Sodium 476mg; Carbohydrates 8g; Fiber 1g (Digestible Carbohydrates 7g); Protein 45g.

Chicken and a Few Duck Dishes

CHICKEN IS THE WONDER AND THE BANE OF EVERY COOK. It's the one bird that can be cooked almost any way, with myriad seasonings, and yet, modern chicken breeding incites tremors of revolution by anyone even remotely concerned with what he consumes. In other words: buy organic free-range chicken if you can. The flavor is far superior to the bland, fatty mass-produced supermarket variety, and the meat, having been spared the advent of growth hormones and genetically-modified feed, is much more healthful.

Throughout the Mediterranean, chicken is a much-adored bird and many people still maintain enough countryside ties to have access now and again to a real free-roaming, yard-strutting bird. There are distinctions in the Mediterranean among young chickens, old hens, and dark-fleshed roosters; it is no accident that one of the Mediterranean's most prized dishes is the French coq au vin—rooster (not hen) in wine—a recipe that finds similar counterparts in many of the greater region's cuisines.

Where once chicken was savored almost exclusively as a festive, or at least Sunday, meal in the Mediterranean, now it is pedestrian fare, sold as takeout at barbecue chicken places and prepared as quick meals in minutes for busy cooks. Perhaps chicken has become so indispensable because it is so versatile, inexpensive, and family-friendly. Every culture in the Mediterranean boasts its classic rendition of roasted chicken. Around the Mediterranean many of those recipes call for similar ingredients, mainly olive oil and lemons, but sometimes also herbs and garlic.

Roasted chicken may be a litmus test for poultry cookery in the region, but the Mediterranean also boasts a wide array of chicken stews and casseroles. The wealth of chicken recipes is good news for low carbers.

The stews are the most interesting and enticing of all the Mediterranean chicken recipes because within their panoply of ingredients one can discern entire cultures. The spices that go into chicken dishes from the eastern Mediterranean and North African countries are blatantly absent from the down-to-earth chicken dishes in Italian cuisine and the more refined chicken dishes of French cuisine. The Spanish tend to favor other birds, mainly game birds, over chicken, but there is still a vast number of Spanish recipes for *pollo,* cooked with garlic, which the Spanish use with abandon, with sherry, red peppers, chorizo, pine nuts, orange sauce, and more. For Greek cooks, chicken and avgolemono, the egg-lemon sauce, are inseparable. My favorite dish among all the recipes that follow is the robust and down-to-earth Circassian chicken, in a version filled with good carbs. One of the most unusual recipes in this collection, for coffee chicken, comes from an Israeli colleague, Daniel Rogov.

I have tried to include recipes here that strive to attain two goals: first, to offer up easy solutions for a quick midweek kind of meal for those watching their carbs, and second, to evoke a sense of the region through one of its most cherished, if common, foods.

Stovetop Chicken Dishes
from the Mediterranean

Chicken Saltimbocca

This classic Roman dish is traditionally prepared with veal cutlets, seasoned with sage, and enriched with prosciutto. Whether made with veal or chicken, its name, which means "hop in the mouth," evokes exactly what saltimbocca is all about—too good to resist. Both easy and elegant, saltimbocca is a dish that can be served for a midweek rush-home-and-cook kind of meal but also one that provides an elegant option for dinner parties.

8 servings

2 pounds chicken cutlets (about 8 cutlets)

8 fresh sage leaves

8 slices prosciutto

2 tablespoons unsalted butter

1 tablespoon olive oil

Salt and freshly ground black pepper

½ cup dry white wine

Place the cutlets between 2 sheets of parchment paper and pound them very thin using a mallet.

Place a sage leaf and then a slice of prosciutto on each pounded cutlet. Roll up and secure closed with a toothpick.

Heat the butter and olive oil in a large nonstick skillet over medium heat. Add the saltimbocca rolls and sauté, turning, to brown lightly on all sides. Season with salt and pepper to taste.

Pour in the wine, lower the heat, cover and simmer for 15 minutes, or until chicken is tender. Remove from the heat and serve, pouring the sauce from the skillet over the chicken.

PER SERVING: Calories 193; Fat 9g (Saturated 3g); Cholesterol 83mg; Sodium 473mg; Carbohydrates 0g; Fiber 0g (Digestible Carbohydrates 0g); Protein 27g.

Braised Chicken Breasts with Eggplant, Tomatoes, and Feta

Stewed vegetables, especially with summer vegetables such as eggplant, green beans, and zucchini, often come in two versions in Greece, a meatless one and a richer, more filling version that may include chicken, lamb, or a number of other meats or fish. This dish is a simplified version of a Greek favorite.

4 servings

2 medium eggplants, trimmed and cut into 1-inch cubes

Salt

4 skinless, boneless chicken breasts, each halved lengthwise

Freshly ground black pepper

4 tablespoons extra virgin olive oil

½ cup chopped red onion

½ cup chopped celery

2 garlic cloves

2 cups drained chopped plum tomatoes

1 teaspoon dried oregano

4 tablespoons crumbled feta

2 tablespoons fresh flat-leaf parsley

Place the eggplant in a colander, salting a little at a time. Let stand in the sink for 1 hour to drain. Rinse and pat dry with paper towels.

Season the chicken with salt and pepper to taste. Heat 2 tablespoons olive oil in a large, wide, nonstick pot or Dutch oven over high heat, add the chicken breasts, and sauté, turning until browned on both sides, about 8 to 10 minutes. Remove the chicken to a platter and set aside.

Using the same skillet, reduce the heat to medium, add the onion and celery, and sauté until translucent, about 5 to 6 minutes. Add 2 tablespoons olive oil, raise the heat, and add the eggplant. Sauté until the eggplant is lightly browned, 4 to 5 minutes. Add the garlic, stir gently for 1 minute, and add the tomatoes.

Transfer the chicken back to the pot, add the oregano, cover, lower the heat, and cook for about 25 minutes, until the chicken is tender. Just before serving, sprinkle in the feta and parsley.

PER SERVING: Calories 360; Fat 19g (Saturated 4g); Cholesterol 81mg; Sodium 480mg; Carbohydrates 18g; Fiber 7g (Digestible Carbohydrates 11g); Protein 31g.

Low-Carb Circassian Chicken

One of the absolute classics of Turkish cuisine, Circassian chicken is enriched with a delicious sauce that calls for a base of stale bread and walnuts, but here a Greek barley rusk, which adds body and texture and fewer carbs, is substituted.

6 servings

2 tablespoons extra virgin olive oil
One 3½-pound chicken, cut into serving-size pieces
Salt and freshly ground black pepper
4 cups chicken broth

The sauce
1 Greek barley rusk (about 3 ounces)
2 tablespoons unsalted butter
1 cup chopped onion
2 garlic cloves, minced
2 teaspoons paprika
½ to 1 teaspoon cayenne pepper
1 cup shelled walnuts
Salt

3 tablespoons chopped flat-leaf parsley, for garnish

Heat the olive oil in a nonstick Dutch oven over high heat and brown the chicken pieces in batches, turning once. Season with salt and pepper to taste. Add the broth, bring to a boil, then reduce the heat. Cover and simmer for about 40 minutes, until the chicken is tender. Remove the chicken, cover, and set aside to cool completely. With the lid off the pot, cook down the pot juices over high heat until they are reduced to 3 cups, about 7 to 10 minutes.

Dip the barley rusk in the broth for a few seconds to soften and break it up into pieces.

Heat the butter in a medium nonstick skillet over medium heat, add the onion, and sauté until wilted, about 4 minutes. Add the garlic, paprika, and cayenne and stir. Remove from heat and set aside to cool.

Place the walnuts in a food processor and process until finely ground and mealy. Break up the barley rusk and add it to the processor. Pulse on and off, taking care not to over-process. Add the onion mixture and 2 cups of the broth. Pulse to combine. Adjust the consistency with additional broth—the sauce should be the consistency of a medium bat-ter—and season with salt.

Shred the chicken and place on a platter. Toss with the sauce, garnish with additional pa-prika and the parsley, and serve.

PER SERVING: Calories 468; Fat 28g (Saturated 7g); Cholesterol 103mg; Sodium 550mg; Carbohy-drates 17g; Fiber 4g (Digestible Carbohydrates 13g); Protein 36g.

Spice Route Chicken

The triad of spices found in this dish—cumin, coriander, and cinnamon—appear in aromatic sauces all over the Mediterranean, but especially in the Eastern Mediterranean and parts of North Africa. This is delicious over simple sautéed or steamed spinach.

6 servings

One 4- to 4½-pound chicken, cut into pieces and skinned

3 tablespoons extra virgin olive oil

Salt and freshly ground black pepper

1 cup chopped red onion

½ cup finely chopped green pepper

½ cup finely chopped red pepper

2 garlic cloves, minced

2 teaspoons ground coriander

1 teaspoon ground cumin

½ teaspoon ground cinnamon

2 bay leaves

2 cups chopped plum tomatoes

2 cups chicken broth

2 tablespoons seedless golden raisins

8 pitted and coarsely chopped Kalamata olives

Wash and pat dry the chicken. Heat the olive oil in a Dutch oven or wide nonstick pot over medium-high heat. Add the chicken, season with salt and pepper, and brown on all sides. You may have to do this in batches. Remove with a slotted spoon. Drain all but 2 tablespoons fat out of the pot. Reduce the heat to medium, add the onions, peppers, and garlic, and cook until wilted, 4 to 5 minutes. Add the coriander, cumin, cinnamon, and bay leaves and stir for 1 minute with a wooden spoon.

Season the chicken with salt and pepper to taste and place it back in the pot. Add the tomatoes and broth. Bring to a boil, reduce the heat, cover, and simmer until the chicken is tender, about 45 minutes.

While the chicken is cooking, plump the raisins in ¼ cup warm water, then drain. Add the raisins and olives to the pot 5 minutes before removing from the heat. Adjust the seasoning with salt and pepper, and serve.

PER SERVING: Calories 342; Fat 18g (Saturated 4g); Cholesterol 105mg; Sodium 415mg; Carbohydrates 9g; Fiber 2g (Digestible Carbohydrates 7g); Protein 36g.

Lemony One-Pot Chicken

Lemon, garlic, and dill give this dish its Greek identity.

6 servings

One 3- to 4-pound chicken, cut into 8 pieces and skinned
2 tablespoons extra virgin olive oil
Salt and freshly ground black pepper
1 large leek, whites and tender part of the greens, coarsely chopped
1 medium fennel bulb, coarsely chopped
2 garlic cloves, minced
½ cup dry white wine
1½ cups chicken broth
½ cup chopped fresh dill
1 large egg, beaten
Juice of 1 large lemon, or more to taste

Wash and pat dry the chicken. Heat the olive oil in a Dutch oven over medium-high heat and brown the chicken on all sides. Season with salt and pepper. You may have to do this in batches. Remove the chicken with a slotted spoon and set aside.

Spoon out all but 2 tablespoons of fat from the pot, reduce the heat to medium, add the leek, fennel, and garlic, and cook until translucent, 5 to 6 minutes. Return the chicken to the pot, season with salt and pepper to taste, and stir gently with a wooden spoon so that the vegetables are distributed all around the chicken pieces. Pour in the wine, and when it steams up, pour in the broth and enough water to barely cover the chicken. Cover and simmer for 45 minutes, or until the chicken is tender. Add the dill 5 to 10 minutes before turning the heat off.

Prepare the egg-lemon sauce: Whisk together the egg and lemon juice in a medium bowl. Take a ladleful of the pot liquid and add it to the egg-lemon mixture in a slow, steady stream, whisking all the while. Repeat with a second ladleful. Pour the mixture over the chicken, tilt the pot back and forth to distribute evenly, and remove from heat. Do not cover the pot. Serve immediately.

PER SERVING: Calories 307; Fat 14g (Saturated 6g); Cholesterol 104mg; Sodium 345mg; Carbohydrates 7g; Fiber 1g (Digestible Carbohydrates 7g); Protein 36g.

Provençal Chicken Stew

Here's an easy, elegant, flavorful chicken recipe inspired from the olive-infused dishes of Southern France.

6 servings

One 4½-pound chicken, cut into 8 pieces and skinned
Salt and freshly ground black pepper
3 tablespoons olive oil
½ cup chopped red onion
4 garlic cloves, minced
3 tablespoons diced lean smoked pork or Canadian bacon
3 cups chopped plum tomatoes, with their juices
2 cups chicken broth
½ cup dry white wine
2 bay leaves
1 scant tablespoon chopped fresh thyme
½ cup Niçoise olives, pitted, rinsed, and drained
½ cup chopped fresh basil

Wash and pat dry the chicken and season with salt and pepper to taste. Heat the olive oil in a Dutch oven or large, wide pot over medium-high heat and brown the chicken in batches, turning to color on all sides. Remove the chicken with a slotted spoon.

Pour off all but 2 tablespoons fat from the pot. Reduce the heat to medium, add the onion, and cook until it starts to turn golden, about 10 minutes. Add the garlic and cook for 1 minute, stirring. Add the smoked pork and cook for about 1 minute.

Place the chicken back in the pot and add the tomatoes, broth, and wine. Raise the heat to high and bring to a boil. Reduce the heat to low, add the bay leaves and thyme, and simmer until the chicken is tender, about 45 minutes. About halfway through cooking the chicken add the olives, and about 5 minutes before removing the pot from the heat, add the basil.

PER SERVING: Calories 391; Fat 21g (Saturated 4g); Cholesterol 121mg; Sodium 834mg; Carbohydrates 8g; Fiber 1g (Digestible Carbohydrates 7g); Protein 42g.

Chicken Fricassee with Carrots, Artichokes, and Herbs

Fricassee refers to many different dishes all over the Mediterranean. In Greece, as in France, a fricassee sauce is always white, although the Greeks use egg and lemon as opposed to heavy cream to achieve the color and velvety texture. In Italy, fricassee refers to a stew of many a different color and flavor. This dish evokes a Greek classic.

6 servings

One 3½- to 4-pound chicken, cut into 8 pieces and skinned

The Marinade
½ cup extra virgin olive oil
6 tablespoons strained fresh lemon juice
1 teaspoon grated lemon zest
2 garlic cloves, smashed
Freshly ground black pepper
1 tablespoon dried mint

2 tablespoons extra virgin olive oil
½ cup chopped leek, whites only
½ cup diced onion
2 large carrots, cut into ½-inch dice
½ cup dry white wine
3 cups chicken broth
6 large artichoke hearts, preferably from fresh artichokes or very good quality frozen, defrosted

The egg-lemon sauce
1 large egg
Juice of 1 large lemon

⅓ cup finely chopped fresh mint

Wash and pat dry the chicken. Whisk together all the marinade ingredients in a stainless steel bowl and toss with the chicken pieces. Cover and refrigerate for 6 to 24 hours. Remove the chicken from the marinade just before cooking and pat dry.

Heat the 2 tablespoons olive oil in a large nonstick pot or Dutch oven over medium-high heat. Season the chicken with salt and pepper and brown, in batches, in the Dutch oven. Remove with a slotted spoon and set aside.

Pour off all but 2 tablespoons of the fat from the pot, reduce the heat to medium, add the leek, onion, and carrots and cook, stirring, until softened, 6 to 7 minutes. Add the chicken to the pot, stir, and pour in the wine. When the wine steams up, add the broth and enough water to barely cover the chicken. Bring to a boil, reduce the heat, partially cover, and simmer until the chicken is tender, about 45 minutes.

About 15 minutes before removing chicken from heat, add the artichoke hearts, mixing gently to cover with the pot liquids. Simmer until the artichoke hearts are fork tender. Remove the chicken and vegetables from the pot and place on a large, deep serving platter. Cover with aluminum foil to keep warm.

Pour the liquid back into the pot and simmer until it is reduced to about 3 cups.

In a medium bowl, whisk together the egg and lemon juice until frothy. Add a ladleful of the pot juices to the egg mixture in a slow, steady stream, whisking all the while. Repeat with another ladleful, then pour the mixture into the pot, tilting it to distribute evenly. Add the mint and remove from the heat. Uncover the chicken, cover with sauce, and serve.

PER SERVING: Calories 347; Fat 18g (Saturated 4g); Cholesterol 128mg; Sodium 189mg; Carbohydrates 11g; Fiber 4g (Digestible Carbohydrates 7g); Protein 34g.

Chicken Smothered with Red Cabbage and Wine

The combination of cabbage and chicken is found in various parts of the Mediterranean. In Northern Greece, for example, there are a handful of similar dishes except the palate of flavors there becomes distinctly Balkan, calling for pickled cabbage as opposed to the sweet red cabbage in this lovely winter dish.

6 servings

1 tablespoon extra virgin olive oil

1 cup finely chopped red onion

2 garlic cloves, smashed

6 cups shredded red cabbage, rinsed and drained

One 4½-pound chicken, cut into 8 pieces and skinned

Salt and freshly ground black pepper

2 tablespoons olive oil

½ cup dry red wine

1 cup chicken broth

Heat the 2 tablespoons extra virgin olive oil in a Dutch oven or large, wide pot over medium heat, add the onion and cook, stirring until wilted and lightly golden, 8 to 10 minutes. Add the garlic and cook for 1 to 2 minutes, stirring. Just as the garlic begins to color, add the cabbage. Cover and cook down until the cabbage is reduced in volume by half.

Meanwhile, wash and pat dry the chicken. Season with salt and pepper to taste. Heat the 2 tablespoons olive oil in a separate large nonstick skillet over medium-high heat and brown the chicken, in batches if necessary. Remove the chicken with a slotted spoon and set aside.

Remove half the cabbage from the pot and set aside. Spread the remaining half evenly over the bottom of the pot. Place the chicken pieces on top and cover with remaining cabbage. Pour in the wine and broth and season with salt and pepper to taste. Cover the pot, reduce the heat to medium-low and simmer until the chicken is tender and falling off the bone and the cabbage almost disintegrated, about 1 hour. Remove from the pot and serve.

PER SERVING: Calories 345; Fat 17g (Saturated 4g); Cholesterol 117mg; Sodium 333mg; Carbohydrates 7g; Fiber 2g (Digestible Carbohydrates 5g); Protein 40g.

Chicken Cacciatore

It seems ironic at best that a dish for the world's most domesticated fowl should be called "hunter's" chicken, which is what cacciatore means in Italian.

6 servings

One 4½-pound chicken, cut into 8 pieces and skinned
Salt and freshly ground black pepper
3 tablespoons olive oil
1 cup finely chopped onion
½ cup coarsely chopped celery
1 large carrot, coarsely chopped
½ cup dry white wine
1 large red pepper, cored, seeded, and coarsely chopped
3 garlic cloves, finely chopped
1 teaspoon fresh rosemary
2 cups chopped plum tomatoes, with their juices

Wash and pat dry the chicken and season with salt and pepper to taste. Heat the olive oil in a large Dutch oven over medium-high heat and brown the chicken, in batches if necessary. Remove the chicken with a slotted spoon and set aside.

Pour off all but 2 tablespoons fat from the pot. Turn the heat back on to medium, add the onion, celery, and carrot, and cook until the onion is lightly browned and the celery is translucent, about 10 minutes. Add the wine, allowing it to steam up. Reduce the heat a little and simmer until the wine is almost completely cooked off.

Add the red pepper, garlic, and rosemary to the pot and cook for 3 to 4 minutes, stirring, until the red pepper softens. Add the tomatoes. Bring to a simmer and place the chicken pieces back in the pot, mixing with a wooden spoon to evenly distribute. Cover, reduce the heat, and simmer gently until the chicken is very tender and falling off the bone, about 50 minutes. Add a little water during cooking if necessary to keep the contents of the pot from drying out. Adjust the seasoning with salt and pepper and serve.

PER SERVING: Calories 345; Fat 17g (Saturated 4g); Cholesterol 116mg; Sodium 327mg; Carbohydrates 8g; Fiber 2g (Digestible Carbohydrates 6g); Protein 39g.

Balsamic-Honey Glazed Chicken Breasts

There are some recipes in this book that are a little more lenient than others with their carb count. This is one of them. But the honey is negligible—just enough to impart the hint of sweetness and to help give this dish its final flavor profile, slightly sweet and sour.

4 servings

2 tablespoons olive oil

4 boneless, skinless chicken breasts

Salt and freshly ground black pepper

1 cup thinly sliced yellow onions

4 garlic cloves, slivered

½ cup pureed fresh or canned tomatoes

½ cup chicken broth or water

4 tablespoons balsamic vinegar

2 teaspoons honey

Heat the oil in a large nonstick skillet over high heat. Season the chicken breasts with salt and pepper, add to the pan, and sauté, turning once, to brown lightly on both sides. Remove the chicken from the skillet and set aside. Pour off all but 2 tablespoons fat from the skillet.

Reduce the heat to low, add the onions and garlic, and cook until wilted, about 6 to 7 minutes. Add the tomato puree and broth. Using a wooden spoon, scrape the bottom of the skillet to gather up any bits of chicken that are stuck to it.

Transfer the chicken breasts back to the skillet. Cover and simmer for 30 minutes, or until the chicken is tender. Remove the chicken breasts to a platter and tent with aluminum foil to keep warm.

Whisk together the vinegar and honey in a small bowl and pour into the pan, stirring. Simmer for 5 to 10 minutes, until the sauce is reduced to about ½ cup. Drizzle the sauce over the chicken and serve.

PER SERVING: Calories 243; Fat 10g (Saturated 2g); Cholesterol 74mg; Sodium 383mg; Carbohydrates 10g; Fiber 1g (Digestible Carbohydrates 9g); Protein 28g.

Pan-Seared Chicken Breasts
with a Variety of Relishes

It might seem odd to suggest a mix-and-match recipe, which indeed this is. I like to make all three relishes with this simple chicken dish and indulge in all of them with forkfuls of the seared chicken.

8 servings

THREE DIFFERENT RELISHES

Tuscan Tomato-Basil Topping

2 medium ripe tomatoes, seeded and diced

1 roasted red pepper in brine, drained and diced

½ cup finely chopped red onion

1 garlic clove, pressed

½ cup finely chopped fresh basil

2 teaspoons balsamic vinegar

Greek Salad Topping

2 medium ripe tomatoes, seeded and diced

1 small fresh chile, seeded and finely chopped

¼ cup finely chopped red onion

¼ cup pitted Kalamata olives

1 scant teaspoon dried oregano

1 tablespoon extra virgin olive oil

1 to 2 teaspoons strained fresh lemon juice

Moroccan Olive, Orange, and Almond Topping

½ cup pitted Moroccan oil-cured olives, coarsely chopped

½ cup pitted green olives, coarsely chopped

½ cup coarsely ground blanched almonds

¼ navel orange, peeled and diced

½ teaspoon ground cumin

½ teaspoon finely grated orange zest

½ teaspoon cayenne pepper

1 tablespoon extra virgin olive oil

The chicken

2 pounds boneless, skinless chicken breasts

Salt and freshly ground black pepper

2 tablespoons olive oil

To prepare any or all of the toppings: Combine all the ingredients for each and allow them to marinate for 1 hour at room temperature. The Tuscan Tomato-Basil Topping and Greek Salad Topping can be made a little further ahead of time and left to marinate in the refrigerator for up to 3 hours.

To make the chicken: Place the chicken breasts between 2 sheets of parchment paper and hammer them with a mallet. Each piece should be about ⅛-inch thick. Season lightly with salt and pepper. Heat the olive oil in a large nonstick skillet over high heat, add the chicken breasts, and sauté for about 3 minutes per side, or until tender and lightly browned. Remove from the heat and serve with any of the above toppings.

PER SERVING: Calories 283; Fat 17g (Saturated 2g); Cholesterol 63mg; Sodium 543mg; Carbohydrates 9g; Fiber 2g (Digestible Carbohydrates 7g); Protein 25g.

Chicken in the Oven

Clay Pot Chicken with Roasted Lemons

This dish takes its cue from Morocco, with a shortcut. Instead of the preserved lemons that are a traditional condiment to Moroccan cuisine, the lemons are roasted to achieve a similar flavor. The clay pot adds another dimension, one of earthiness that speaks of the entire Mediterranean. If you don't have an ovenproof clay baking dish, use any earthenware, ceramic, or ovenproof glass baking dish and bake as directed. If you have an enamel or cast-iron Dutch oven, then prepare the dish in one pot.

6 servings

The lemons

1 large lemon, cut into 6 wedges

1 tablespoon olive oil

Salt

The chicken

One 4-pound chicken

Salt and freshly ground black pepper

2 tablespoon olive oil

3 tablespoons small capers, rinsed and drained

½ cup cracked green Greek or Sicilian olives, pitted

3 garlic cloves, smashed

¼ cup chopped flat-leaf parsley

½ cup dry white wine

Preheat the oven to 325°F. Line a small baking sheet with parchment paper. Place the lemon wedges on the sheet, brush with the olive oil, and sprinkle with salt. Roast for about 1 hour, until the lemon wedges begin to dry out and brown around the edges.

Meanwhile, wash and pat dry the chicken and season with salt and pepper. Heat the olive oil in a nonstick pot or Dutch oven over high heat and brown the chicken, turning to color all over. Transfer the chicken and pot juices to a clay baking dish large enough to hold the chicken. If you're using a Dutch oven, you can bake the chicken directly inside it.

Remove the lemons from the oven. Raise the heat to 350°F. Place the lemon wedges around the chicken. Sprinkle the capers, olives, garlic, and parsley around the chicken. Pour in the wine and ½ cup water. Cover the clay pot with its lid or with aluminum foil and bake the chicken for 50 minutes to 1 hour, until tender, basting occasionally. Remove and serve on a platter with the lemons, capers, olives, garlic, and herbs around the chicken.

PER SERVING: Calories 492; Fat 34g (Saturated 8g); Cholesterol 134mg; Sodium 924mg; Carbohydrates 4g; Fiber 1g (Digestible Carbohydrates 3g); Protein 43g.

Under the Skin Herb-Roasted Chicken

The herbs inserted under the skin of the chicken impart their flavor as the bird roasts. Rosemary, thyme, oregano, fennel, and, of course, garlic make for a spectrum of flavors savored all over the Mediterranean world, but this particular dish takes its cue from the sunny tables of Provence. The dish is traditionally made with butter, not olive oil, under the skin.

6 servings

One 4½-pound roasting chicken
2 tablespoons extra virgin olive oil
2 large garlic cloves
1 tablespoon chopped fresh rosemary
1 tablespoon chopped flat-leaf parsley
1 tablespoon chopped fresh thyme
1 tablespoon chopped fresh oregano
1 scant teaspoon fennel seeds
Salt and freshly ground black pepper
1 onion, peeled and quartered
1 small fennel bulb, trimmed and quartered
1 carrot, sliced
6 garlic cloves
1½ cups chicken broth
½ cup dry white wine
1 tablespoon whole-wheat flour

Wash the chicken inside and out and pat dry. Preheat the oven to 400°F. Position the rack in the center of the oven. Using a mortar and pestle pound 2 tablespoons extra virgin olive oil with 2 garlic cloves, the rosemary, parsley, thyme, oregano, fennel seeds, and a little salt and pepper to make a thick paste. Sprinkle the inside of the chicken with a little salt and pepper.

Starting at the neck end, slide your fingers under the skin of the chicken's breast and thighs to make a pocket. Rub the flesh of the chicken with the herb paste. Season the chicken with salt and pepper on the outside. Place the onion, fresh fennel, carrot, and remaining 4 garlic cloves inside the chicken's cavity and scatter what doesn't fit in the pan, drizzling with a little more extra virgin olive oil. Tie the legs together with kitchen twine. Roast the chicken, uncovered, for 30 minutes, until browned.

Pour the broth and wine into the pan and continue roasting the chicken for another 30 to 40 minutes, basting it with the pan juices every 10 minutes or so. Remove from the oven. Transfer the chicken to a serving platter and cover with aluminum foil to keep warm.

Place the roasting pan on top of the stove, over 2 burners if necessary, at medium-high heat. Bring to a simmer. Scrape the browned bits of chicken and vegetables off the bottom of the pan. Pour the liquid into a measuring cup and spoon off the fat that rises to the top, reserving 1 tablespoon.

Heat the reserved tablespoon of fat in a medium saucepan over medium heat, add the flour, and cook 2 to 3 minutes. Do not brown. Add the pan juices to the pot and bring to a simmer. Simmer until thickened, stirring, 5 to 6 minutes. Season with salt and pepper and serve the sauce with the chicken. Remove the skin from the chicken before serving.

PER SERVING: Calories 305; Fat 15g (Saturated 4g); Cholesterol 117mg; Sodium 140mg; Carbohydrates 2g; Fiber 0g (Digestible Carbohydrates 2g); Protein 39g.

Spiced Chicken Baked Under a Brick

I found this intriguing, deliciously succulent dish in a cookbook by Waldy Malouf, chef at Beacon restaurant in New York and adapted it adding some of my own spices. The result is a juicy, intensely flavored chicken dish that is surprisingly easy to prepare. My recipe tester, Brigitte, adds her own comment on the title. She baked the chicken under a brick . . . found at a construction site. Note that this recipe requires planning ahead so the chicken can marinate in the spice rub.

6 servings

1 whole roasting chicken, about 4½ pounds, halved and breastbone removed
   (ask the butcher to do this)
1 tablespoon cumin seeds
½ tablespoon fennel seeds
½ tablespoon coriander seeds
4 allspice berries
15 black peppercorns
2 garlic cloves
2 teaspoons turmeric
1 teaspoon ground ginger
½ teaspoon paprika
½ teaspoon cayenne pepper
1 teaspoon kosher salt
3 tablespoons extra virgin olive oil
1 lemon, quartered
2 tablespoons chopped flat-leaf parsley, for garnish

Rinse and pat dry the chicken. Remove the skin. Using a mortar and pestle, pulverize all the spices and salt together with 1 tablespoon olive oil to form a paste. You can also pulverize the whole spices first in a spice grinder and then mix them with the ground spices and olive oil. Rub the spice mixture all over the top of the chicken. Wrap the chicken tightly in plastic wrap and allow it to marinate in the spice rub in the refrigerator for 12 to 24 hours.

Remove the chicken from the refrigerator 1 hour before roasting.

Wrap 2 bricks with aluminum foil. Place in the oven together with a heavy, ungreased roasting pan or large cast-iron or enamel skillet. Turn the oven on to the highest setting, 500°F if possible. Heat the pan and the bricks for 15 minutes.

Unwrap the chicken and rub each piece with 1 tablespoon olive oil. Press the pieces flat with the palm of your hand. Wearing heavy-duty oven mitts, carefully remove the pan from the oven and place the chicken halves in it, skin-side down. Place a brick on top of each chicken half and roast at for 30 minutes. The chicken will be highly flavorful and succulent. Remove from the oven and serve garnished with lemon wedges and parsley.

PER SERVING: Calories 324; Fat 17g (Saturated 4g); Cholesterol 3mg; Sodium 431mg; Carbohydrates 3g; Fiber 1g (Digestible Carbohydrates 2g); Protein 38g.

Lebanese Roasted Chicken

Garlic, lemon, and cumin are the triad of flavors that speak of the eastern Mediterranean.

6 servings

The marinade

Juice of 2 large lemons

2 tablespoons extra virgin olive oil

6 garlic cloves, smashed

1 tablespoon chopped fresh thyme

1 teaspoon paprika

1 teaspoon ground cumin

½ teaspoon cayenne pepper

One 4-pound roasting chicken, cut into 8 pieces and skinned

Salt and freshly ground black pepper

Lemon wedges, for garnish

2 tablespoons fresh chopped parsley, for garnish

Whisk together the lemon juice, olive oil, garlic, thyme, paprika, cumin, and cayenne in a large bowl. Toss with the chicken, cover, and refrigerate for 8 to 24 hours, turning occasionally.

Remove the chicken from the refrigerator 1 hour before baking it so it's at room temperature.

Preheat the oven to 450°F. Transfer the chicken to a roasting pan. Season with salt and pepper to taste. Pour the marinade over the chicken and roast for 15 minutes. Reduce the oven temperature to 375°F and continue roasting for another 30 to 40 minutes, until tender and golden, basting with the pan juices every 10 to 15 minutes. Remove the chicken to a platter, spoon the pan juices over the chicken halves, garnish with lemon wedges and parsley, and serve.

PER SERVING: Calories 316; Fat 10g (Saturated 2g); Cholesterol 135mg; Sodium 120mg; Carbohydrates 3g; Fiber 0g (Digestible Carbohydrates 3g); Protein 50g.

Roast Chicken Stuffed with Spinach, Wild Rice, Walnuts, and Feta

My Greek roots come through in this dish. One of the classics of Greek peasant cooking is the spinach-rice pilaf that is often served with feta cheese. I have reworked it, using wild rice and walnuts, and instead of serving it as an accompaniment outside *the bird, I cook it on the inside as a stuffing. There is a similar, traditional stuffed turkey dish, filled with spinach and a slew of herbs, from Naxos.*

6 servings

One 4½-pound roasting chicken
¼ cup wild rice
Salt
½ pound fresh spinach, trimmed
3 tablespoons extra virgin olive oil
I small red onion, finely chopped
3 tablespoons ground walnuts
¼ teaspoon ground nutmeg
¼ cup crumbled Greek feta
I tablespoon seedless golden raisins
Freshly ground black pepper
½ cup dry white wine

Wash and pat dry the chicken. Set aside.

Rinse the wild rice and bring it to a boil in a medium pot of ample salted water over high heat. Reduce the heat and simmer for about 25 minutes, until al dente. Remove from the heat and drain into a colander.

Steam the spinach. Remove from the heat, cool, and coarsely chop. Drain the spinach very well in a colander for I hour, squeezing to get as much of the liquid out as possible. You should have about ½ cup spinach.

Heat I tablespoon olive oil in a nonstick skillet over medium heat add the onion and sauté until wilted, about 5 minutes.

Combine the spinach, onion, wild rice, walnuts, nutmeg, feta, and raisins in a medium bowl. Season with salt and pepper to taste. Add I tablespoon olive oil and mix well. Preheat the oven to 375°F.

Wash and pat dry the chicken. Rub it with the remaining tablespoon olive oil and season with salt and pepper to taste. Fill the cavity of the chicken with the spinach mixture. Place the chicken on a rack in a shallow baking pan and roast for 15 minutes. Reduce the oven temperature to 350°F, pour the wine over the chicken, and add ½ water to the pan. Continue roasting the chicken for about 45 minutes, until browned and the juices run clear when the chicken is pierced in the thigh. Baste 2 or 3 times with the drippings as the chicken roasts. Remove, cool slightly, spoon out the filling, and serve the chicken with the vegetables on the side. Remove skin from the chicken before serving.

PER SERVING: Calories 390; Fat 20g (Saturated 5g); Cholesterol 123mg; Sodium 427mg; Carbohydrates 10g; Fiber 2g (Digestible Carbohydrates 8g); Protein 42g.

Israeli Orange Chicken

This is a popular holiday dish in Israel, and one that appears in many different versions.

8 servings

One 4- to 5-pound roasting chicken
½ orange, unpeeled
Salt and freshly ground black pepper
One 1-inch piece ginger root, minced
1 small cinnamon stick
1 small whole orange, peeled
1 medium yellow onion, sliced
2 tablespoons fresh orange juice
2 teaspoons honey
⅓ cup dry white wine

Preheat the oven to 350°F. Lightly oil a medium baking dish.

Wash and pat dry the chicken. Rub the orange half on the outside of the chicken, squeezing its juice and pulp all over. Season with salt and pepper to taste and rub with half the ginger. Place the remaining ginger, cinnamon stick, and whole orange inside the chicken's cavity. Place in a roasting pan and sprinkle with the onion slices.

Roast the chicken for 30 minutes. Whisk together the orange juice, honey, and wine. Brush the chicken with this mixture every 10 to 15 minutes, for another 30 to 40 minutes, until the chicken is tender and its juices run clear when pierced in the thigh. Remove from oven, remove the orange and cinnamon stick from the cavity. Remove skin, carve, and serve.

PER SERVING: Calories 307; Fat 14g (Saturated 3g); Cholesterol 116mg; Sodium 307mg; Carbohydrates 5g; Fiber 0g (Digestible Carbohydrates 5g); Protein 38g.

Israeli Coffee Chicken

This has got to be one of the most unique recipes in the whole Mediterranean! According to the Israeli food journalist Daniel Rogov, this dish did not originate in Israel but in the Jewish homes of Iran and Iraq in the late nineteenth century. The dish was introduced to Israel when Irani and Iraqi Jews immigrated during the 1940s and 1950s and has remained popular primarily as a home-cooked dish. Rogov says he knows of only one restaurant that ever served the dish and that was Eucalyptus in Jerusalem, which is now closed.

6 to 8 servings

4 pounds bone-in chicken breasts or mixed chicken parts (breasts, thighs, legs), skinned

1 cup decaffeinated black coffee

2 tablespoons tomato paste

2 tablespoons low-sodium soy sauce

2 tablespoons fresh strained lemon juice

2 tablespoons olive oil

2 tablespoons honey

Rinse and pat dry the chicken and place in a lightly oiled shallow baking dish. Preheat the oven to 350°F.

Combine all the remaining ingredients in a small saucepan over high heat and bring to a boil. Reduce the heat and simmer for about 8 to 10 minutes, to reduce and thicken slightly. Pour the coffee mixture over the chicken pieces, tossing to coat. Bake, uncovered, for 45 minutes to 1 hour, basting occasionally with the pan juices, until the chicken is tender. Remove from the oven and serve.

PER SERVING: Calories 305; Fat 10g (Saturated 2g); Cholesterol 120mg; Sodium 311mg; Carbohydrates 8g; Fiber 0g (Digestible Carbohydrates 8g); Protein 45g.

Moroccan Spiced Chicken Stew
with Chickpeas and Almonds

This dish is traditionally prepared with smen, *a strong-flavored Moroccan butter, and preserved lemons. I replace the smen with a combination of butter and olive oil and use fresh lemons in lieu of the traditional Moroccan salted, preserved lemons.*

6 servings

One 4½-pound chicken, cut into 8 pieces and skinned
1 lemon, halved
Salt and freshly ground black pepper

The Spice Paste
4 garlic cloves
2 tablespoons chopped flat-leaf parsley
One ½-inch piece ginger, peeled and minced
½ teaspoon turmeric
2 tablespoons extra virgin olive oil

The Broth
1 tablespoon unsalted butter
1 tablespoon olive oil
1 cup finely chopped onion
1 to 1½ cups chicken broth
½ teaspoon saffron, crushed
1 cinnamon stick
½ cup blanched almonds
½ cup canned chickpeas, drained and rinsed
1 tablespoon strained fresh lemon juice

Wash and pat dry the chicken pieces. Rub the chicken pieces with lemon, vigorously squeezing the lemon into the flesh of the chicken. Season with salt and pepper to taste.

Using a mortar and pestle or small food processor, pulverize the garlic, parsley, ginger, turmeric, and extra virgin olive oil until the mixture is a dense paste. Rub the chicken pieces with the spice paste, place in a shallow bowl, cover with plastic wrap, and refrigerate for 24 hours.

Remove the chicken from the refrigerator 1 hour before cooking. Melt the butter and olive oil in a large nonstick pot over low heat, add the onion and cook until lightly golden, 10 to 12 minutes. Raise the heat a little, add the chicken pieces, and brown lightly on all sides. Pour in 1 ½ cups of the broth. Raise the heat to high, bring to a boil, then reduce the heat, add the saffron and cinnamon, and simmer, covered, for about 1 hour, until the chicken is practically falling off the bone. Add remaining broth during cooking to keep the chicken moist. Remove the chicken to a platter and tent with foil to keep warm.

Add the almonds to the pot liquid, along with the chickpeas. Raise the heat and simmer for 8 to 10 minutes, until the sauce thickens. Add the lemon juice, adjust the seasoning with salt and pepper, pour the sauce over the chicken pieces, and serve.

PER SERVING: Calories 432; Fat 25g (Saturated 5g); Cholesterol 121mg; Sodium 281mg; Carbohydrates 10g; Fiber 3g (Digestible Carbohydrates 7g); Protein 42g.

Rosemary-Orange Duckling

Duck began its Mediterranean journey as an exotic treat, savored by the Romans, who liked to stuff a whole chicken inside a whole duck and with that fill the cavity of a whole goose. Today, duck is decidedly more prosaic, mainly because most of what one finds in the Mediterranean as well as in the United States is farm-raised, not wild, hence much more accessible.

6 servings

One 5-pound duckling, neck and giblets removed
Salt and freshly ground black pepper
3 garlic cloves, pressed
2 teaspoons dried rosemary
1 orange, quartered
1 slim leek, trimmed and cut into 4 pieces
2 tablespoons dry red wine
2 tablespoons fresh orange juice
1 tablespoon balsamic vinegar
½ teaspoon brown sugar

Start 1 day before cooking the duck: Wash and pat the duck dry and season with salt and pepper to taste. Using a mortar and pestle, crush the garlic and rosemary to a paste and rub it all over the duck, inside and out. Refrigerate the duck, uncovered, for 1 day. It will absorb the seasoning, its skin will dry out, and the resulting bird, once roasted, will be crispy on the outside.

Preheat the oven to 375°F. Prick the skin of the duck with the tines of a fork, taking care not to puncture its flesh. Stuff the duck's cavity with the orange and leek. Place breast-side down on a rack in a shallow baking pan in the middle of the oven and roast for 1 hour. Turn the duck over to roast on the other side for about 1 more hour, or until the juices run clear when the duck is pierced. Remove from the pan and tent with aluminum foil for about 15 minutes before carving.

Pour out all but 2 tablespoons of the drippings from the pan. Place the pan on the stove-top over medium heat and scrape up the bits that are stuck to the bottom. Pour in the wine. As soon as it sizzles, pour in the orange juice and vinegar. Sprinkle in the sugar and cook the pan juices for a minute or 2, until thickened. Remove the sauce, pour it into a small bowl, and serve with the duck.

PER SERVING: Calories 408; Fat 30g (Saturated 15g); Cholesterol 115mg; Sodium 285mg; Carbohydrates 2g; Fiber 0g (Digestible Carbohydrates 2g); Protein 29g.

Peppery Lemon Duck with Roasted Garlic

6 servings

One 5-pound duckling
Salt and freshly ground black pepper
2 garlic cloves, pressed
3 tablespoons black peppercorns
Grated zest of 2 lemons
1 whole head garlic
Juice of 3 large lemons
Juice of 2 large juice oranges
½ cup dry white wine

Start 1 day before cooking the duck: Wash and pat the duck dry and season with salt and pepper to taste. Using a mortar and pestle, crush the garlic, peppercorns, and lemon zest to a paste and rub it all over the duck, inside and out. Refrigerate the duck, uncovered, for 1 day. It will absorb the seasoning, its skin will dry out, and the resulting bird, once roasted, will be crispy on the outside.

Preheat the oven to 375°F. Prick the skin of the duck with the tines of a fork, taking care not to puncture its flesh. Fill the duck's cavity with the whole garlic head. Combine the lemon and orange juices in a medium bowl.

Place the duck breast-side down on a rack in a shallow baking pan in the middle of the oven. Pour the juice over it and roast for 1 hour, basting every 15 to 20 minutes, until the exposed half is nicely browned. Turn the duck over and continue roasting another hour, basting every 15 to 20 minutes. The duck is ready when its juices run clear when the duck is pierced. Remove from the pan and tent with aluminum foil for about 15 minutes before carving. Remove the garlic from the duck's cavity before carving.

Prepare a gravy from the pan juices: Pour out all but 2 tablespoons of the drippings from the pan. Place the pan on the stovetop over medium heat and scrape up the bits that are stuck to the bottom. Pour in the wine. As soon as it sizzles, reduce the heat and simmer for 5 to 6 minutes, until thickened. Remove the sauce, pour it into a small bowl, and serve with the duck.

PER SERVING: Calories 447; Fat 30g (Saturated 10g); Cholesterol 115mg; Sodium 288mg; Carbohydrates 11g; Fiber 1g (Digestible Carbohydrates 10g); Protein 30g.

The Sacrificial Lamb

N O MEAT, INDEED, PERHAPS NO OTHER RAW INGREDIENT save for olive oil, seems as fundamental to the Mediterranean table as lamb. If pork breeds contention, lamb breeds unity. Muslims, Jews, and Christians alike all eat lamb. Religious, cultural, and ethnic differences from Istanbul to Madrid disappear before a plate of grilled lamb, for not only do most people savor the meat; every culture around the basin has recipes for it grilled or roasted. Even more than olive oil, lamb is the one food that everyone, everywhere in the Mediterranean can relate to, a food with a formidable staying power. Lamb was the food of ancient sacrificial offerings and legendary heroic feasts. Today, throughout the Mediterranean, it is both festive and pedestrian, the stuff of holiday feasts and street food alike.

From the kebabs of Turkey to the souvlaki and Paschal lamb of Greece to the Easter lamb of Italy and France and the tagines of

North Africa, traditional lamb recipes abound. I find it intriguing to survey the differences from one country to the next, as lamb, one of the region's culinary unifiers, is also a good mirror of how certain flavors define certain cultures. In Greece, for example, lamb is almost always seasoned with a lot of garlic, oregano, and lemon juice, although regional recipes abound for sweeter lamb stews, flavored with cinnamon, tomatoes, and quince, or with spring vegetables such as artichokes. Egyptians make a lemony lamb stew with peas. Ground lamb is used much more in the cuisines of Turkey and the Middle East than it is in the kitchens of Greece, Italy, France, and Spain. For the Turks, beyond their famed street food, kebabs and gyro, lamb and yogurt is the perfect match. The French have the most delicate way with lamb, particularly with their gorgeous roasted racks and saddles of lamb. In Italy, lamb bridges an East-West sensibility. Italian lamb dishes, such as lamb shanks with beans and simple herb-crusted roasted legs, tend to be earthy and robust. Morocco boasts a great wealth of lamb dishes, from fragrant tagines to kefta to lamb, with a carb-counter's taboo, couscous.

Lamb also provides much of the prized offal meats that Mediterranean peoples have been feasting on long before such foods made headlines. Sweetbreads, liver, and tripe almost always come from lamb in this part of the world. Cooks in the Mediterranean share yet another point of view when it comes to how they look upon lamb. For most people the best lamb is the youngest, spring-born, milk-fed lamb.

In a nod to the needs of American cooks, most of the lamb recipes in the following pages call for lamb chops, which are easy to find and easy to cook. I have included a handful of more festive dishes, for leg of lamb prepared in various ways, knowing that adherents to a low-carb way of life also cook for friends now and again. Lamb, the quintessential Mediterranean meat, provides a perfect main course.

Three Lamb Kebabs

Skewered lamb, the quintessential meat dish of the Eastern Mediterranean, comes in infinite variations. Herbs are always a part of the dish, either as part of the marinade or as the skewer itself, as in the whole rosemary sprigs that are used as skewers in the Rosemary-Threaded Lamb Kebabs.

Rosemary-Threaded Lamb Kebabs

Rosemary and lamb go hand in hand. Rosemary "skewers" can be found in many supermarkets. Serve these kebabs with a simple green salad and fried potato skins.

6 servings

½ cup dry red wine

4 tablespoons extra virgin olive oil

3 garlic cloves, minced

2 teaspoons finely chopped rosemary

Salt and freshly ground black pepper

3 pounds boneless leg of lamb, trimmed and cut into 1½-inch cubes

6 medium red onions, each cut into 6 wedges

Twelve 8-inch sprigs fresh rosemary

In a medium bowl, whisk together the wine, olive oil, garlic, rosemary, and salt and pepper to taste. Toss the lamb cubes in the marinade, cover, and marinate for 1 hour at room temperature, or up to 6 hours refrigerated. Preheat the broiler. Place the oven rack 6 inches from the heat source.

Thread the lamb and onion wedges in alternating pieces onto the rosemary skewers, always starting with the root end of the rosemary and working the pieces onto the sprig from the bottom up, in the direction of the bristles. Broil the lamb, brushing it with the marinade, for 10 to 12 minutes total, for medium-rare. Serve immediately.

PER SERVING: Calories 305; Fat 15g (Saturated 4g); Cholesterol 98mg; Sodium 223mg; Carbohydrates 8g; Fiber 2g (Digestible Carbohydrates 6g); Protein 32g.

Grilled Skewered Lamb
with Mint and Garlic Pesto

Here is a Greek twist on pesto.

8 servings

The Lamb

3 pounds boneless leg of lamb, trimmed and cut into 1½-inch cubes

4 tablespoons extra virgin olive oil

Salt

1 teaspoon freshly ground black pepper

3 large garlic cloves, slivered

The Pesto

2 tablespoons blanched almonds

2 garlic cloves

2 bunches fresh mint, leaves only, coarsely chopped

¼ cup grated Greek feta

3 tablespoons extra virgin olive oil

2 tablespoon fresh lemon juice

Freshly ground black pepper

Salt

Eight 12-inch metal or wooden skewers

Place the lamb in a large bowl and toss with the olive oil, salt, pepper, and garlic. Cover and marinate for 1 hour at room temperature or up to 6 hours refrigerated. Bring to room temperature before cooking.

If using wooden skewers, soak them in water for 30 minutes before using. Preheat the broiler. Place the oven rack 6 inches from the heat source.

Pulverize the almonds and garlic in a food processor. Add the mint and pulse on and off to mix. Add the feta, olive oil, lemon juice, and pepper to taste. Pulse to combine. Season with salt to taste. Set the pesto aside at room temperature for 30 minutes to 1 hour before serving.

Thread the lamb pieces onto the skewers. Arrange the skewers in a single layer on a baking sheet and brush with the marinade. Season with salt to taste. Broil the lamb for 10 to 12 minutes total, turning once for medium-well. Remove from the oven and serve with the pesto.

PER SERVING: Calories 349; Fat 23g (Saturated 5g); Cholesterol 102mg; Sodium 422mg; Carbohydrates 3g; Fiber 1g (Digestible Carbohydrates 2g); Protein 33g.

Spicy Lamb Kebabs

This is a dish that comes from one of my favorite Athenian tavernas, Valentina.

8 servings

3 pounds boneless leg of lamb, trimmed and cut into 2-inch cubes
5 tablespoons extra virgin olive oil
Freshly ground black pepper
1 to 2 teaspoons cayenne pepper, plus more for dusting
6 tablespoons sour cream
3 medium red onions, sliced into paper-thin rings
4 tablespoons finely chopped flat-leaf parsley
Lemon wedges, for garnish

Eight 8-inch metal skewers

Place the lamb pieces in a large bowl and toss with 3 tablespoons olive oil, the black pepper, and cayenne. Cover and marinate for 1 hour at room temperature or up to 6 hours refrigerated. Bring to room temperature before cooking.

Preheat the broiler and place the oven rack 6 inches from the heat source.

Thread the lamb pieces onto the skewers. Arrange the skewers in a single layer on a baking sheet and brush with the marinade. Broil the lamb for 10 to 12 minutes total, turning once, for medium-rare.

While the lamb is broiling, combine the sour cream and remaining 2 tablespoons olive oil. Remove the kebabs to a platter or to individual plates. Top the kebabs with the raw onion rings, parsley, and a dusting of cayenne. Serve immediately with the sour cream and lemon wedges on the side.

PER SERVING: Calories 279; Fat 14g (Saturated 5g); Cholesterol 102mg; Sodium 83mg; Carbohydrates 4g; Fiber 1g (Digestible Carbohydrates 3g); Protein 32g.

Lamb Baked in Parchment Paper

This is one of the classics of the Eastern Mediterranean and a great dish to present to company.

4 servings

2 pounds boneless leg of lamb, cut into 2-inch cubes

2 tablespoons extra virgin olive oil

4 tablespoons fresh lemon juice

4 garlic cloves, thinly sliced

2 teaspoons dried oregano

2 teaspoons dried thyme

Salt and freshly ground black pepper

4 ounces Greek feta or Parmesan, cut into 1-inch cubes

1 large ripe tomato, cut into 8 slices

1 lemon, cut into 8 slices

In a large bowl, combine the lamb cubes, olive oil, lemon juice, garlic, oregano, thyme, and salt and pepper to taste. Toss well. Cover and let stand at room temperature for 1 hour, or in the refrigerator for up to 3 hours. If refrigerating, bring the meat up to room temperature before baking.

Preheat the oven to 350°F.

Divide the meat mixture among four 18- by 18-inch pieces of parchment paper. Divide the cheese cubes among each parcel and top each little mound of filling with 2 tomato slices and 2 lemon slices. Bring up the sides of the parchment and fold over to form a package.

Place the parcels in a shallow baking pan and sprinkle with a little water. Bake for 2 hours. Remove the parcels from oven, place on individual serving plates, and open carefully, as the steam that escapes will be very hot. Serve.

PER SERVING: Calories 385; Fat 19g (Saturated 9g); Cholesterol 155mg; Sodium 494mg; Carbohydrates 5g; Fiber 1g (Digestible Carbohydrates 4g); Protein 46g.

Grilled Lamb Chops Stuffed with Mushrooms, Onions, and Herbs

Lamb chops are fairly common fare, whether during the week or on weekends. By stuffing them, they become decidedly more festive. The mushrooms help keep them moist, too.

4 servings

Four 1-inch-thick lamb chops, trimmed
⅔ cup dry red wine
4 tablespoons extra virgin olive oil
3 garlic cloves, smashed
5 to 6 juniper berries, crushed
Freshly ground black pepper

The Stuffing
1 tablespoon olive oil
4 scallions, trimmed and chopped
2 large garlic cloves, minced
½ pound mushrooms, stems removed and caps cleaned and sliced thin
  (reserve the stems for another use)
Salt and freshly ground black pepper
1 scant teaspoon dried oregano or thyme
4 tablespoons chopped flat-leaf parsley

Rinse and pat dry the lamb. Using a sharp knife, make a pocket in the thickest part of the lamb chops. Whisk together the wine, extra virgin olive oil, garlic, juniper berries, and pepper to taste in a large bowl and toss the lamb chops in the mixture. Cover and marinate for 1 hour at room temperature or up to 6 hours in the refrigerator.

About 20 minutes before cooking the meat, preheat the broiler or grill, setting the rack about 6 inches from the heat source, and prepare the stuffing: Heat the olive oil in a medium skillet over medium heat, add the scallions and garlic and sauté until translucent, about 4 minutes. Add the mushrooms and sauté until the mushrooms no longer exude liquid and the skillet is relatively dry, about 8 to 10 minutes. Season with salt and pepper to taste and add the oregano and parsley. Allow to cool slightly.

Remove the lamb chops from the marinade and pat dry. Reserve the marinade.

Fill the lamb chops with several spoonfuls of the mushroom mixture and press to close. Broil or grill the chops, turning once and brushing occasionally with the marinade, for about 8 minutes for rare, 12 to 14 minutes for medium-rare, and about 18 minutes for well done. Serve immediately. If any of the mushroom mixture is left, heat it gently a few minutes before removing the chops from the broiler and serve it spooned around the meat.

PER SERVING: Calories 278; Fat 22g (Saturated 4g); Cholesterol 44mg; Sodium 346mg; Carbohydrates 5g; Fiber 1g (Digestible Carbohydrates 4g); Protein 16g.

Balsamic-Glazed Lamb Chops
with Red Pepper Pesto

An Italian-inspired recipe that is great to look at and redolent of one robust flavor after another.

4 servings

The Red Pepper Pesto
3 red peppers, roasted, peeled, and seeded
2 garlic cloves
1 cup chopped fresh basil
2 tablespoons extra virgin olive oil
2 teaspoons balsamic vinegar
Salt and freshly ground black pepper

2 teaspoons finely chopped fresh rosemary
1 teaspoon dried thyme
Salt and freshly ground black pepper
4 garlic cloves, minced
Four 1-inch-thick lamb chops, trimmed
2 tablespoons extra virgin olive oil
1 red onion, finely chopped
⅓ cup balsamic vinegar
½ cup chicken broth

Place the roasted peppers, garlic, basil, olive oil, and vinegar in a food processor and pulse on and off for a few seconds. The pesto should be a little chunky. Season with salt and pepper to taste.

Using a mortar and pestle, pound the rosemary, thyme, salt and pepper to taste, and 2 of the garlic cloves together. Rinse and pat dry the lamb. Rub the lamb chops all over with the mixture.

Heat the olive oil in a large, heavy nonstick skillet over high heat until nearly smoking. Sear the lamb chops, in 2 batches if necessary, 3 to 4 minutes per side for medium-rare, 5 to 6 minutes per side for medium, and about 8 minutes per side for well-done. Remove and set aside, covered, to keep warm.

Lower the heat a little add the onion and remaining 2 cloves garlic and sauté in the same skillet for about 2 minutes, or until wilted. Add the vinegar and broth. Raise the heat, bring to a boil, then reduce the heat and simmer for about 5 minutes, until reduced by half. Season with salt and pepper to taste. Spoon the sauce over the chops on a platter or on individual plates and serve with the red pepper pesto on the side.

PER SERVING: Calories 290; Fat 19g (Saturated 4g); Cholesterol 44mg; Sodium 644mg; Carbohydrates 16g; Fiber 4g (Digestible Carbohydrates 12g); Protein 16g.

Seared Lamb Chops
with Lemon-Caper Sauce

Lamb is the natural backdrop for all sorts of other seasonings, from rosemary to oregano to garlic and lemon. Here, it is paired with both lemons and capers, and with no small share of herbs.

4 servings

2 bay leaves

2 teaspoons grated lemon zest

3 garlic cloves, smashed

2 teaspoons dried oregano or marjoram

I teaspoon freshly ground black pepper

3 tablespoons extra virgin olive oil

Four I-inch-thick lamb chops, trimmed

The sauce

4 scallions, chopped

3 garlic cloves, finely chopped

2 teaspoons whole-wheat flour

⅓ cup dry white wine

I cup chicken or vegetable broth

2 teaspoons grainy Dijon mustard

Dash of cayenne pepper

¼ cup light cream

2 teaspoons strained fresh lemon juice

2 tablespoons capers, rinsed, drained, and chopped

Using a mortar and pestle, pound the bay leaves, lemon zest, garlic, oregano, pepper, and I tablespoon olive oil together into a paste. Rinse and pat dry the lamb. Rub the lamb chops with the mixture and wrap tight, individually, in plastic wrap. Let stand at room temperature for 1 hour. Remove the plastic wrap.

Heat 1 tablespoon olive oil in a heavy nonstick skillet over high heat. Sear the lamb chops, in 2 batches if necessary, for 3 to 4 minutes per side for medium-rare, 5 to 6 minutes per side for medium, and about 8 minutes per side for well-done. Remove and set aside, covered, to keep warm.

Using the same skillet, reduce the heat to medium, heat the remaining tablespoon olive oil, add the scallions and garlic, and sauté for 6 to 7 minutes, until soft. Sprinkle with the flour. Cook, stirring, for another 2 minutes. Pour in the wine. When the wine steams up, pour in the chicken broth. Simmer until slightly thickened, 6 to 7 minutes. Add the mustard and cayenne and stir. Pour in the heavy cream and heat it through. Stir in the lemon juice and capers. Place the lamb chops on a platter or on individual plates and spoon the sauce evenly over each chop.

PER SERVING: Calories 230; Fat 14g (Saturated 5g); Cholesterol 55mg; Sodium 213mg; Carbohydrates 8g; Fiber 2g (Digestible Carbohydrates 6g); Protein 16g.

Greek-Style Butterflied Leg of Lamb
with Walnut–Grape Leaf–Ouzo Pesto

Lamb is the de facto festive meat from Turkey to Morocco, so I could not pass over the importance of roasted lamb in this book. This recipe is not exactly traditional—it was born out of two sources. The first is Periyali, a Greek restaurant in New York City that served something similar on its menu many, many years ago; the second is grape-leaf pesto, a new Greek product a friend developed several years ago. I have done my own share of tinkering and offer up the results.

8 servings

10 grape leaves in brine

6 tablespoons extra virgin olive oil

1 medium red onion, finely chopped

1 medium fennel bulb, finely chopped

6 garlic cloves, minced

2 tablespoons ouzo or other anise-flavored liqueur

1 bunch parsley, leaves only, chopped

½ cup chopped fresh mint

⅔ cup walnuts

½ cup crumbled Greek feta

Salt and freshly ground black pepper

One 8-pound leg of lamb, boned, and butterflied (or 4 to 5 pounds boneless), trimmed of fat

1 teaspoon black peppercorns

2 teaspoons dried oregano

½ cup dry red wine

2 cups beef broth

1 teaspoon fennel seeds

2 teaspoons corn starch, dissolved in 2 tablespoons cold water

Rinse the grape leaves under running water. Bring a medium pot of water to a rolling boil and blanch the grape leaves for 5 minutes. Remove to a colander and rinse again. Trim off the stems and coarsely chop the leaves.

Heat 2 tablespoons olive oil in a large, heavy skillet over medium heat, add the onion, fresh fennel and, 2 garlic cloves and sauté for about 5 minutes, until softened. Pour in the ouzo carefully and let it evaporate.

Combine the grape leaves, onion-fennel mixture, parsley, mint, walnuts, and feta in a food processor and pulse on and off to combine. Add 2 tablespoons olive oil to moisten the mixture and season with salt and pepper to taste.

Preheat the oven to 325°F. Rinse and pat dry the lamb. Place it boned side up on a work surface and season it with salt and pepper to taste. Spread the filling evenly over the surface of the lamb, leaving a 1-inch border around the edges. Beginning with one of the short sides, roll up the lamb jelly-roll fashion and tie it tightly with kitchen string.

Using a mortar and pestle, ground 1 teaspoon black peppercorns, the oregano, remaining 4 cloves garlic, and remaining 2 tablespoons olive oil. Season the lamb with salt and rub the herb mixture all over the surface of the lamb. Place the lamb in a roasting pan and roast for approximately 20 minutes per boneless pound (for medium-rare), or about 1¾ hours.

Remove the lamb to a platter while making the sauce. Skim off the fat from the pan drippings and discard. Place the roasting pan on the stovetop over medium-high heat. Add the wine, scrape up any charred bits from the bottom of the pan, and simmer, stirring, until the mixture is reduced by half. Strain the mixture through a sieve and pour the liquid into a saucepan. Add the broth, fennel seeds, and any juices that have oozed out of the lamb on the platter. Boil the mixture until reduced by half. Whisk in the cornstarch mixture and simmer for about 2 minutes, until thickened.

Remove the strings from around the lamb, carve into ¼-inch slices, and serve with the sauce.

PER SERVING: Calories 473; Fat 29g (Saturated 7g); Cholesterol 138mg; Sodium 515mg; Carbohydrates 6g; Fiber 2g (Digestible Carbohydrates 4g); Protein 46g.

Greek Lamb with Spinach, Herbs, and Feta

This festive lamb preparation was often a Sunday special when I was growing up, and it's one I continue to make for my own kids.

8 servings

1 pound fresh flat-leaf spinach, trimmed

4 tablespoons extra virgin olive oil

3 large garlic cloves, minced

3 scallions, finely chopped

½ cup snipped fresh dill

⅓ cup chopped fresh mint

¼ pound Greek feta, crumbled

One 8-pound leg of lamb, boned and butterflied (or 4 to 5 pounds boneless), trimmed of fat

Salt and freshly ground black pepper

2 teaspoons dried oregano

2 teaspoons dried thyme

2 teaspoons crumbled dried rosemary

1 large red onion, cut into thick slices

½ cup dry red wine

2 cups beef broth

1 teaspoon cornstarch dissolved in 2 tablespoons cold water

Chop the spinach coarsely and wash it very well in several baths of cold water. Drain. Place the spinach in a heavy saucepan, and steam it in the water clinging to the leaves, over medium heat, covered, for 3 to 5 minutes, or until wilted. Drain the spinach in a colander, let it cool slightly, and squeeze it between the palms of your hands to get out as much of the water as possible.

Heat 2 tablespoons olive oil in a large skillet over medium heat, add the garlic and scallions and cook until wilted and lightly colored, 4 to 5 minutes. Add the spinach and sauté for another minute or 2, until any remaining water has evaporated. Allow the spinach to cool in the skillet. Add the dill, mint, and feta.

Preheat the oven to 350°F.

Rinse and pat dry the lamb. Arrange the lamb on a work surface, boned side up, and season it with salt and pepper to taste. Spread the spinach-feta mixture evenly over the lamb, leaving a 1-inch border around the edges. Beginning with the short side closest to you, roll it up jelly-roll fashion and tie it tightly with kitchen string or fit an elastic meat net over it.

Transfer the lamb to a roasting pan and rub the remaining 2 tablespoons olive oil all over. Using a mortar and pestle, pound together the oregano, thyme, rosemary, 1 tablespoon salt, and pepper to taste and rub the mixture all over the lamb. Roast the lamb for 30 minutes. Sprinkle the onion over and around the lamb and continue roasting another 1 to 1¼ hours (a total of 20 minutes cooking time for each pound of boneless meat), or until a meat thermometer registers 135°F for medium-rare. Transfer the lamb to a cutting board and let it rest for 20 minutes before carving.

While the lamb is resting, make the gravy: Skim the fat from the pan drippings and set the roasting pan on the stovetop, over high heat. Add the wine, deglaze the pan, scraping up the brown bits, and boil the mixture until it is reduced by half. Strain through a fine sieve into a saucepan. Add the broth, ½ cup water, and any juices that have accumulated on the cutting board. Bring to a boil, reduce the heat to medium, and simmer until the liquid is reduced to about 2 cups. Stir the cornstarch mixture, add it to the hot liquid, whisking, and simmer for another 2 to 3 minutes, until slightly thickened. Season with salt and pepper, strain into a gravy boat, and serve with the lamb.

PER SERVING: Calories 379; Fat 18g (Saturated 7g); Cholesterol 143mg; Sodium 1,288mg; Carbohydrates 6g; Fiber 2g (Digestible Carbohydrates 4g); Protein 46g.

Leg of Lamb with Yogurt-Spice Marinade

In Turkey, highly aromatic and spiced lamb is often served with a dollop of thick sheep's milk yogurt. Here, the yogurt is used in the marinade.

8 servings

2 tablespoons coriander seeds

2 tablespoons fennel seeds

2 tablespoons cumin seeds

I tablespoon coarsely ground black pepper

½ teaspoon turmeric

½ teaspoon cayenne pepper

6 garlic cloves, minced

¼ cup extra virgin olive oil

⅓ cup plain whole yogurt

Salt

One 8-pound leg of lamb, boned and butterflied (or 4 to 5 pounds boneless), trimmed of fat

Grind the coriander, fennel seeds, and cumin together in a spice mill or with a mortar and pestle. Place in a medium bowl and add the black pepper, turmeric, cayenne, garlic, olive oil, yogurt, and salt to taste.

Rinse and pat dry the lamb. Place the lamb in the roasting pan and brush the marinade all over its surface. Cover and refrigerate for at least I hour or up to 3 hours.

Preheat the oven to 350°F and roast the lamb, basting every 15 minutes or so with the pan juices, for about 45 minutes for rare, about 50 minutes for medium-rare, and about I hour for well done. Remove the meat from the oven and let it rest for 20 minutes before serving. Slice and serve, drizzled with the pan juices, if desired.

PER SERVING: Calories 367; Fat 19g (Saturated 5g); Cholesterol 131mg; Sodium 255mg; Carbohydrates 4g; Fiber 2g (Digestible Carbohydrates 2g); Protein 43g.

Boneless Leg of Lamb with Olive Paste and Rosemary

Leg of lamb invites a holiday aura. This dish is comfortingly simple to make and may be served with equal ease on holidays and ordinary days alike.

8 servings

1 cup pitted Kalamata olives or ⅔ cup store-bought Kalamta olive paste
5 large garlic cloves
2 tablespoons dried rosemary
Salt and freshly ground black pepper
¼ cup extra virgin olive oil
One 8-pound leg of lamb, boned (or 4½ to 5 pounds boneless)

Preheat the oven to 350°F.

Pound the olives or olive paste, garlic, rosemary, and salt and pepper to taste together with a mortar and pestle and gradually add the olive oil in a thin stream, pounding all the while, until the mixture becomes a paste.

Rinse and pat dry the lamb. Place the lamb in a baking pan boned side up and rub the olive paste generously all over. Roast the lamb, basting every 15 minutes or so with the pan juices, for about 45 minutes for rare, about 50 minutes for medium-rare, and about 1 hour for well done. Remove the meat from the oven and let it rest for 20 minutes before serving. Slice and serve, drizzled with the pan juices, if desired.

PER SERVING: Calories 424; Fat 24g (Saturated 6g); Cholesterol 147mg; Sodium 533mg; Carbohydrates 2g; Fiber 0g (Digestible Carbohydrates 2g); Protein 47g.

Roasted Lamb Shoulder
with Moroccan Spices

Here is a holiday lamb dish that is often cooked by Moroccan Jews.

8 servings

1 lamb shoulder, about 5 pounds, trimmed
2 garlic cloves, minced
Salt and freshly ground black pepper
3 tablespoons olive oil
2 scant teaspoons ground ginger
1 tablespoon dried mint
⅔ cup dry white wine
One 1-inch strip orange zest

Wash and pat dry the lamb. Preheat the oven to 400°F.

Using a mortar and pestle, pound the garlic, salt and pepper to taste, olive oil, the ginger, and mint to a paste. Rub the lamb shoulder all over with the mixture. Place in a baking pan and roast for 30 minutes.

Meanwhile, bring the wine and orange zest to a boil in a small saucepan over medium heat. Reduce the heat and simmer for 5 minutes.

Open the oven door, pour the wine and zest over the lamb, reduce the heat to 350°F and continue roasting basting every 15 to 20 minutes with the pan juices, for 1 to 1½ hours, until the lamb is done. It takes about 20 minutes per pound for medium rare. Remove the lamb from the oven and let it rest for 15 to 20 minutes before slicing, then serve.

PER SERVING: Calories 457; Fat 28g (Saturated 10g); Cholesterol 169mg; Sodium 260mg; Carbohydrates 1g; Fiber 0g (Digestible Carbohydrates 1g); Protein 48g.

The Ubiquitous Pig and a Few Beef Dishes

I F LAMB IS THE MEDITERRANEAN'S GREAT CARNAL UNIFIER, pork is the meat of contention, separating Christians from Muslims and Jews. Throughout most of the European Mediterranean, though, no other meat is as important. Pork provided agricultural families with yearlong sustenance; to this day in villages all over the Mediterranean, people engage in the yearly festive pork slaughter, which usually occurs around Christmas and provides nourishment through Easter.

The wealth of charcuterie, from Iberian ham to prosciutto di Parma to sausages of every stripe, is one of the greatest aspects of the Mediterranean table. Charcuterie is so much a way of life, especially in Italy and Spain, that it is considered a separate category of food, not meat per se. In Spain, ham is sold in almost every food shop. The vast array of Mediterranean charcuterie is one of the region's greatest gifts to low-carbers, too.

Pork in other forms enjoys a prominent place on the tables of all of Europe's Mediterranean countries and among the Christian populations in the Middle East and North Africa. The Greeks tend to like their pork dishes stewed, although grilled pork, especially as street food (souvlaki, gyro, and the like) is also savored. Pork tenderloin is a favorite cut in Greece and something one often finds on restaurant menus, stuffed or braised with wine, with vegetables, nuts, and dried fruit. Easier to cook cuts, such as pork chops, tend to be grilled in the Greek kitchen. The crown roast is the king of the Italian festive table, usually seasoned with garlic, olive oil, and rosemary. Shoulder is another cut favored for large, more festive meals, and one that is found throughout the Mediterranean, from Greece to Spain. Pork shoulder is also the recommended cut for many stews.

I have culled from the repertoire of Mediterranean pork dishes recipes that are best suited to North American kitchens. There are several recipes, for example, for pork chops, because they are easy to find, easy to cook, and inexpensive. The aim of this book is to provide ideas for dinner every night of the week, and chops are a good carte blanche for experimenting with all sorts of different flavor combinations from the greater Mediterranean. Pork also lends itself to one of the Mediterranean's most traditional ways of cooking—braising—and I've included a handful of simple recipes for braised pork. I have included two stews and one sausage dish, using my favorite of all Mediterranean sausages, the robust Spanish chorizo, again, easy to find in North America.

Beef, I must admit, is not one of my favorite foods, perhaps reflecting my background as a Greek cook. I will surely indulge in a great grilled steak now and again stateside, but I don't much like cooking it. And I don't believe one needs to turn to a Mediterranean cookbook to learn about grilling or barbecuing beef. I do offer up one steak recipe, though not a grilled one, but for the French classic, steak au poivre, seared in a stovetop skillet. It is also one of the few recipes in this book that call for cream. I wanted the recipes to reflect the way I like to eat, and cream isn't a frequent indulgence. And, finally, because I love all the great daubes of France, I have included a classic one here, a slow-cooked beef stew that communicates the essential message about all Mediterranean food: that it should be patiently and slowly cooked and should rely on the best seasonal ingredients available.

Baked Pork Chops over Tarragon Apples

Inspired from an Asturian dish, chuletas de cerdo Asturias.

4 servings

1 tablespoon extra virgin olive oil

Four 1-inch-thick center-cut pork chops, trimmed of fat

Salt and freshly ground white pepper

1 small green apple (about 4 ounces), peeled, cored, halved, and cut into ⅛-inch slices

2 teaspoons dried tarragon

1 scant teaspoon nutmeg

1 scant teaspoon cinnamon

½ cup chicken broth

2 tablespoons unsweetened apple juice

1 tablespoon unsalted butter

Preheat the oven to 350°F.

Heat the olive oil in a heavy, nonstick skillet over high heat and sear the pork chops for 1 to 2 minutes per side, until deeply browned. Season with salt and pepper, cover, and set aside.

Oil an ovenproof glass baking dish large enough to hold the chops snugly.

Place half the apple slices on the bottom of the baking dish. Sprinkle with ½ teaspoon each of tarragon, nutmeg, and cinnamon. Season lightly with pepper. Place the pork chops over the apples. Season with a little more nutmeg, cinnamon, and another ½ teaspoon tarragon. Cover with the remaining apples and season again with nutmeg, cinnamon, the remaining tarragon, and pepper.

Warm the broth and apple juice in a small pot over medium heat. Pour over the pork chops and add the butter. Cover and bake for 35 to 45 minutes, until the chops are tender. Remove from the oven and serve immediately.

PER SERVING: Calories 231; Fat 13g (Saturated 5g); Cholesterol 71mg; Sodium 351mg; Carbohydrates 6g; Fiber 1g (Digestible Carbohydrates 5g); Protein 23g.

Braised Pork Chops with Rosemary, Fennel, Roasted Red Peppers, and Orange

I often prepare this for casual dinner parties. The Spanakopita Soufflé on page 34 looks great and works well with this dish.

4 servings

The Sauce

2 teaspoons fresh rosemary leaves

1 scant teaspoon fennel seeds

1 tablespoon extra virgin olive oil

4 garlic cloves, minced

3 large red peppers, roasted, peeled, cored, seeded, and chopped

2 tablespoons small capers, drained

Three 1-inch strips orange zest

2 teaspoons balsamic vinegar

Salt and freshly ground black pepper

2 tablespoons olive oil

Four ¾- to 1-inch-thick, center-cut pork chops trimmed of fat

½ cup dry white wine

Salt and freshly ground black pepper

Using a mortar and pestle, grind the rosemary and fennel seeds together and set aside. Heat 1 tablespoon of the extra virgin olive oil in a medium nonstick skillet over medium heat, add the garlic, and sauté for 1 to 2 minutes, until soft. Add the peppers and stir to combine. Add the capers, ground herbs, orange zest, vinegar, and salt and pepper to taste. Cover and cook for 6 to 7 minutes, for the flavors to meld. Remove from the heat and set aside.

Heat the remaining olive oil in a large heavy skillet large enough to hold the pork chops in 1 layer over high heat. Sear the chops for 1 to 2 minutes per side to brown deeply. Pour in the wine. As soon as it evaporates, season the chops with salt and pepper to taste, turning, and add the pepper mixture to the skillet over and all around the chops. Cover, reduce the heat, and cook for about 45 minutes, until the chops are tender. Remove from the heat and serve immediately.

PER SERVING: Calories 321; Fat 21g (Saturated 5g); Cholesterol 66mg; Sodium 468mg; Carbohydrates 10g; Fiber 3g (Digestible Carbohydrates 7g); Protein 24g.

Skillet Braised Pork Chops
with Mushroom Sauce

The Italians are masters of braised pork dishes. Similar dishes exist in the Italian repertoire that call for other, more exotic mushrooms, such as porcini and morels, which could certainly be used here, too.

4 servings

Four 1-inch-thick center-cut pork chops

8 slices prosciutto, trimmed of fat and coarsely chopped

2 teaspoons chopped fresh rosemary

2 teaspoons chopped fresh thyme

2 tablespoons grated Parmesan

1 tablespoon plus 2 teaspoons olive oil

Salt and freshly ground black pepper

2 garlic cloves, minced

¾ pound white mushrooms, trimmed and sliced

2 teaspoons whole-wheat flour

½ cup dry white wine

1 cup chicken broth

Using a sharp boning or paring knife, make a pocket-like incision in each of the pork chops on the inner, boneless side.

Combine the prosciutto, rosemary, thyme, Parmesan, 1 teaspoon olive oil, and salt and pepper to taste in a small bowl. Stuff the pork chops with the mixture, dividing it evenly among the 4 chops. Press closed so that the filling doesn't spill out.

Heat 1 teaspoon olive oil in a large, heavy skillet over medium heat. Add the garlic and sauté for 1 minute, until soft. Add the mushrooms, cover, and cook until they have lost about a third of their volume, about 6 to 7 minutes. Sprinkle with the flour and cook, stirring, for 1 minute. Pour in the wine and broth. Raise the heat, bring to a boil, then immediately reduce the heat to low. Simmer for 5 minutes, or until the juices begin to thicken. Season lightly with salt and pepper.

In a separate large, nonstick skillet, heat the remaining 1 tablespoon olive oil over high heat and sear the pork chops, turning to color them a deep brown on both sides, 1 to 2 minutes per side. Pour the mushroom mixture all around the chops. Cover, reduce the heat, and simmer until the chops are tender, about 40 minutes. Remove from the heat and serve immediately.

PER SERVING: Calories 300; Fat 16g (Saturated 5g); Cholesterol 91mg; Sodium 960mg; Carbohydrates 6g; Fiber 1g (Digestible Carbohydrates 5g); Protein 34g.

Pork Medallions Marinated
with Olives and Orange

The flavor of the pork improves if it marinates for at least six, but better yet twenty-four, hours. Serving various meats and fish over light vegetable and legume broths is something I picked up from a friend and chef here in Athens. Spinach and black-eyed peas are often stewed together in Greece. In this version, the flavors are clean and light; all the heartiness comes from the intensely flavored medallions.

This dish makes a great dinner party entrée. The black-eyed pea and spinach mixture can be prepared separately and served with a simple piece of grilled or pan-fried white-fleshed fish, too, or with grilled steak.

6 servings

The Marinade

Juice of ½ orange

I heaping tablespoon Kalamata olive tapenade

I large garlic clove, minced

2 tablespoons extra virgin olive oil

2 tablespoons dry red wine

One 1½-pound pork loin, trimmed and cut into 1-inch-thick pieces

The Vegetable-Bean Broth

¾ cup dried black-eyed peas

I bay leaf

3 cilantro sprigs

3 parsley sprigs

I garlic clove, smashed but left whole

2 to 3 fennel fronds

Salt and freshly ground black pepper

3 tablespoons extra virgin olive oil

½ medium onion, thinly sliced

½ medium fennel bulb, thinly sliced

2 garlic cloves, slivered

1½ cups defrosted, well-drained frozen chopped spinach or ½ pound fresh spinach,
    steamed, chopped, and drained

Salt and freshly ground white pepper

½ to 1 teaspoon red pepper flakes, to taste

2 tablespoons red wine vinegar

Combine the orange juice, tapenade, minced garlic, 2 tablespoons olive oil, and wine in a large bowl. Add the pork medallions, toss well, cover, and refrigerate for 3 to 24 hours.

Place the black-eyed peas with enough water to cover by 1½ inches in a medium saucepan to a boil over high heat. Drain into a colander, and place back in the pot with fresh water, again enough to cover by 1½ inches, and place over high heat. Add the bay leaf, cilantro and parsley sprigs, whole garlic clove, and fennel fronds. Bring to a boil, then reduce the heat and simmer, uncovered, until almost tender, about 30 minutes. Season with salt and pepper to taste a few minutes before removing from the heat.

Meanwhile, heat 1 tablespoon olive oil in a large, heavy skillet over medium heat. Add the onion, fennel, and garlic slivers and stirring, and sauté until glossy and soft, about 5 minutes. Add the spinach. Season with salt and white pepper to taste and sprinkle in the hot pepper flakes. Reduce the heat to low, cover, and cook over until the spinach is wilted. When the black-eyed peas are almost done and have absorbed nearly all their liquid (there should be a little left in the pot), remove from the heat. Remove and discard the cilantro and parsley sprigs, bay leaf, and whole garlic clove. Pour the contents of the pot into the skillet, mix well, cover, and simmer another 10 to 12 minutes, until black-eyed peas are soft.

Heat 1 tablespoon olive oil in a heavy nonstick skillet, add the pork medallions, and sear on both sides. Lower the heat a little and continue cooking for a total of 8 to 10 minutes, until the pork is cooked through but still tender. Remove. Drizzle the vinegar and remaining 1 tablespoon olive oil into the black-eyed pea and spinach mixture.

Place about 1 cup of the black-eyed pea mixture in a soup bowl and place 2 pork medallions on top. Serve hot.

PER SERVING: Calories 316; Fat 16g (Saturated 4g); Cholesterol 64mg; Sodium 366mg; Carbohydrates 15g; Fiber 4g (Digestible Carbohydrates 11g); Protein 28g.

Easy Braised Pork Chops with Sage Butter, Garlic, and Tomatoes

Sage, butter, and garlic are one of the many flavor trinities for pork in the Mediterranean. This dish, like most of the pork dishes in this book, takes its cue from the aromatic pork cookery of Italy.

4 servings

2 tablespoons unsalted butter

Four ¾- to 1-inch-thick center-cut pork chops, trimmed of fat

2 garlic cloves, slivered

6 fresh sage leaves or 3 dried leaves

1 teaspoon fresh rosemary

Salt and freshly ground black pepper

1 cup coarsely chopped canned plum tomatoes

1 tablespoon balsamic vinegar

Heat the butter in a heavy skillet large enough to fit the chops in 1 layer over medium heat. When the butter bubbles—but before it burns—add the chops. Sear for 1 to 2 minutes on each side, or until they are a deep chestnut-brown color.

Add the garlic, sage, and rosemary and shake the pan back and forth for the flavors to work their way under and around the meat. Season the meat with salt and pepper to taste, turning to flavor both sides. Add the tomatoes, distributing them evenly around and over the chops. Drizzle in the balsamic vinegar. Cover the pan, reduce the heat to low, and braise the chops for 45 minutes to 1 hour, until tender. Remove from the heat and serve immediately.

PER SERVING: Calories 213; Fat 12g (Saturated 6g); Cholesterol 78mg; Sodium 448mg; Carbohydrates 3g; Fiber 0g (Digestible Carbohydrates 3g); Protein 23g.

Pork Stewed with Niçoise Olives and Green Beans

Green beans and protein have been a mainstay in Mediterranean stovetop cookery for centuries. By combining vegetables and protein such as meat or fish, home cooks could stretch a meal.

6 servings

1 tablespoon olive oil

2 pounds boneless pork shoulder, trimmed and cut into 2-inch cubes

1 large red onion, chopped

4 garlic cloves, minced

1½ cups chopped plum tomatoes

1½ cups chicken broth

½ cup dry white wine

1 teaspoon dried thyme, crumbled

1 teaspoon dried oregano, crumbled

1 pound green beans, trimmed

6 sun-dried tomatoes, plumped in warm water for 1 hour

8 Niçoise olives

3 tablespoons finely chopped flat-leaf parsley

Heat the olive oil in heavy, wide pot or Dutch oven over medium-high heat. Brown the pork in the oil, stirring occasionally, for 8 to 10 minutes. Remove the pork with a slotted spoon, transfer to a plate, and set aside for a few minutes.

Reduce the heat to medium-low, add the onions to the same pot, and cook until very soft, about 12 to 15 minutes. Add the garlic and cook, stirring for 2 to 3 minutes, until soft.

Return the pork to the pot. Pour in the tomatoes, broth, wine, thyme, and oregano. Raise the heat and bring to a boil, then reduce heat to medium-low and simmer, partially covered, for 1 hour. Add the green beans to the pot and toss to combine. Continue cooking another 25 to 30 minutes, until tender.

Remove the sun-dried tomatoes from the water and cut into ¼-inch strips. Add to the pot along with their soaking liquid. Continue cooking another 10 to 15 minutes, until most of the liquid evaporates. Add the olives, season with salt and pepper to taste, stir gently, and cook for 5 more minutes, to warm through. Remove from the heat, stir in the parsley, and serve.

PER SERVING: Calories 340; Fat 15g (Saturated 5g); Cholesterol 99mg; Sodium 332mg; Carbohydrates 13g; Fiber 3g (Digestible Carbohydrates 10g); Protein 37g.

Sausage and Seafood Stew with Peppers, Olives, and Tomatoes

Sausage and pepper stews abound, from Greece to Portugal. This dish combines treasures from field, garden, and sea. Try serving it with a small portion of wild rice (a cooked ½ cup portion contains 18 grams of carbs) or with a ½ cup serving of brown rice (23 grams of carbs).

8 servings

1 tablespoon extra virgin olive oil

1 small red onion, thinly sliced

2 garlic cloves, minced

1 medium fennel bulb, halved and cut into ½-inch dice

1 small red pepper, cored, seeded, and cut into ½-inch dice

1 small green pepper, cored, seeded, and cut into ½-inch dice

½ pound sausage, trimmed and cut into ¼-inch dice

2 large ripe tomatoes, peeled, seeded, and chopped, with their juices

½ cup dry white wine

1 cup fish broth or bottled clam juice

1 pound littleneck or other small clams, scrubbed

1 pound unshelled mussels, debearded and scrubbed

½ cup Kalamata olives, pitted and coarsely chopped

3 tablespoons finely chopped flat-leaf parsley

Heat the olive oil in a large, deep skillet or wide, shallow pot over medium heat, add the onion, garlic, fennel, and peppers, and sauté until softened, 5 to 6 minutes. Add the sausage and stir to coat with oil. Add the tomatoes. Bring the mixture to a boil and add the wine. Raise the heat to high and return to a boil. Reduce the heat to low and cover. Simmer until the pot juices are reduced by half, about 10 minutes.

Pour in the fish broth. Raise the heat to high and add the clams and mussels. Cover, reduce the heat to medium-high, and cook until the clams and mussels open, 9 to 12 minutes. Discard any that do not open. Five minutes before removing from heat, add the olives and stir to combine. Just before removing from the heat, stir in the parsley. Serve hot.

PER SERVING: Calories 221; Fat 16g (Saturated 5g); Cholesterol 33mg; Sodium 590mg; Carbohydrates 8g; Fiber 2g (Digestible Carbohydrates 6g); Protein 12g.

A Simple French Country Beef Stew

On a long country weekend with friends many years ago, I made a beef stew recipe from Patricia Well's classic book, Bistro Cooking. It was one of the easiest and most delicious dishes I have ever made, and I have been making it ever since, with various kinds of meat such as lamb and pork and a few of my own seasoning preferences. The stew is essentially a variation of a classic Provençal daube, replete with orange rind and wine, although the latter has been reduced here. This is a great Sunday afternoon lunch dish, especially in the winter. You just have to plan ahead from Friday, leaving the meat to marinate and giving yourself a little time to chill it and skim off the fat that rises and settles on the surface.

Daubes and other beef stews are traditionally served with noodles or mashed or boiled potatoes. Dishes with rich sauces call out for some kind of starch. You could serve these with a very small portion—not more than a cup—of whole-wheat pasta, which has a carb content of about 39 grams. It would be a splurge . . .

6 servings

3 pounds stewing beef, cut into 1½-inch cubes

2 large red onions, coarsely chopped

4 garlic cloves, smashed

2 large carrots, cut into ½-inch rounds

1 celery stalk, trimmed and coarsely chopped

1 small fennel bulb, trimmed and coarsely chopped

1 scant tablespoon dried thyme or ¼ cup chopped fresh thyme

½ cup chopped flat-leaf parsley

2 large bay leaves, cracked

10 to 15 whole black peppercorns

Salt

Two 1-inch strips orange zest

1 cup dry red wine

2 cups beef broth

Start 2 days before serving. On the first day, combine all the ingredients in a large, non-reactive stewing pot or Dutch oven and refrigerate for 24 hours.

The next day, heat the stew over low heat until it begins to simmer. Keep covered and simmer over very low heat for 3½ to 4 hours, until the meat is very tender. Remove from the heat, cool to room temperature, and refrigerate another 12 to 24 hours. The fat will rise to the top and solidify in the refrigerator. Skim the fat off with a large spoon. Return the stew pot to the stove and bring to a simmer over low heat, just to heat through, about 15 to 20 minutes. Remove from the heat, adjust the seasonings with salt and pepper, remove the bay leaves, and serve.

PER SERVING: Calories 374; Fat 16g (Saturated 6g); Cholesterol 141mg; Sodium 467mg; Carbohydrates 9g; Fiber 2g (Digestible Carbohydrates 7g); Protein 46g.

Steak au Poivre

I have purposely avoided using heavy cream to any great length in this book because my intent is to highlight dishes from around the Mediterranean that rely less on butter and cream and more on the region's wealth of vegetables. But there are a few indulgences here and there, and this recipe is one of them. This is a great dish to prepare for company. Serve it with something light, like a green salad.

2 servings

1 tablespoon black peppercorns

1 teaspoon white peppercorns

1 teaspoon dried green peppercorns

2 teaspoons fennel seeds

2 boneless shell steaks (about ¾ pound each)

2 tablespoons olive oil

Salt

3 tablespoons light cream

1 tablespoon brandy

In a mortar and pestle or spice grinder, pound or pulverize the peppercorns and fennel seeds. Spread the spice mixture on a sheet of wax paper or on a large plate. Pat the steaks dry and press both sides of each steak into the mixture to coat.

Heat the olive oil in a large, heavy nonstick skillet over medium heat until hot but not smoking and sear the steaks, about 4 minutes per side for medium-rare. Season with salt, remove from the skillet to a large plate, and tent with foil.

Spoon off the excess fat from skillet and add the cream and brandy. Bring to a boil, then reduce the heat to low, and simmer for 1 to 2 minutes, scraping up any browned bits from the bottom of the skillet. The sauce should be thick and creamy. Season with salt to taste, pour over the steaks, and serve.

PER SERVING: Calories 594; Fat 37g (Saturated 12g); Cholesterol 164mg; Sodium 149mg; Carbohydrates 5g; Fiber 2g (Digestible Carbohydrates 3g); Protein 57g.

Index